BLACKWELL'S

UNDERGROUND CLINICAL VIGNETTES

CLINICAL SCIENCE COLOR ATLAS, STEPS 2 & 3

BLACKWELL'S

UNDERGROUND CLINICAL VIGNETTES

CLINICAL SCIENCE COLOR ATLAS, STEPS 2 & 3

VIKAS BHUSHAN, MD
University of California, San Francisco, Class of 1991
Series Editor, Diagnostic Radiologist

VISHAL PALL, MBBS
Government Medical College, Chandigarh, India, Class of 1996
Series Editor, U. of Texas, Galveston, Resident in Internal Medicine & Preventive Medicine

TAO LE, MD
University of California, San Francisco, Class of 1996

YI-MENG YEN, MD, PHD
University of California Los Angeles, Resident in Orthopaedic Surgery

JORDAN GELLER, MD
Cedars-Sinai Medical Center, Los Angeles, Resident in Internal Medicine

SRISHTI GUPTA, MD, MPP
Harvard Medical School, Class of 2003

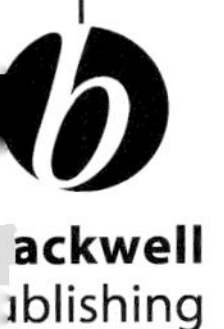

ackwell
ublishing

CONTRIBUTOR

Sonal Shah, MD
Ross University, Class of 2000

FACULTY REVIEWER

Vipal Soni, MD
University of Southern California, Resident in Dermatology

Blackwell Publishing, Inc., 350 Main Street, Malden, Massachusetts 02148-5018, USA
Blackwell Publishing Ltd, 9600 Garsington Road, Oxford OX4 2DQ, UK
Blackwell Science Asia Pty Ltd, 550 Swanston Street, Carlton South, Victoria 3053, Australia

03 04 05 06 5 4 3 2 1

ISBN: 1-4051-0384-1
Blackwell's Undergeround Clinical Vignettes: Basic Science Color Atlas, Steps 2 & 3

Acquisitions: Laura DeYoung
Development: Amy Nuttbrock
Production: Lorna Hind and Shawn Girsberger
Cover design: Leslie Haimes
Interior design: Shawn Girsberger
Typesetter: TechBooks, in Pennsylvania
Printed and bound by Capital City Press, in Vermont

For further information on Blackwell Publishing, visit our website: www.blackwellpublishing.com

Notice:
The indications and dosages of all drugs in this book have been recommended in the medical literature and conform to the practices of the general community. The medications described do not necessarily have specific approval by the Food and Drug Administration for use in the diseases and dosages for which they are recommended. The package insert for each drug should be consulted for use and dosage as approved by the FDA. Because standards for usage change, it is advisable to keep abreast of revised recommendations, particularly those concerning new drugs.

ACKNOWLEDGMENTS

Throughout the production of this book, we have had the support of many friends and colleagues. Special thanks to our support team including Anu Gupta, Andrea Fellows, Anastasia Anderson, Srishti Gupta, Mona Pall, Jonathan Kirsch and Chirag Amin. For prior contributions we thank Gianni Le Nguyen, Tarun Mathur, Alex Grimm, Sonia Santos and Elizabeth Sanders.

We have enjoyed working with a world-class international publishing group at Blackwell Science, including Laura DeYoung, Amy Nuttbrock, Lisa Flanagan, Shawn Girsberger, Lorna Hind and Gordon Tibbitts. For help with securing images for the entire series we also thank Lee Martin, Kristopher Jones, Tina Panizzi and Peter Anderson at the University of Alabama, the Armed Forces Institute of Pathology, and many of our fellow Blackwell Science authors.

For submitting comments, corrections, editing, proofreading, and assistance across all of the vignette titles in all editions, we collectively thank:

Tara Adamovich, Carolyn Alexander, Kris Alden, Henry E. Aryan, Lynman Bacolor, Natalie Barteneva, Dean Bartholomew, Debashish Behera, Sumit Bhatia, Sanjay Bindra, Dave Brinton, Julianne Brown, Alexander Brownie, Tamara Callahan, David Canes, Bryan Casey, Aaron Caughey, Hebert Chen, Jonathan Cheng, Arnold Cheung, Arnold Chin, Simion Chiosea, Yoon Cho, Samuel Chung, Gretchen Conant, Vladimir Coric, Christopher Cosgrove, Ronald Cowan, Karekin R. Cunningham, A. Sean Dalley, Rama Dandamudi, Sunit Das, Ryan Armando Dave, John David, Emmanuel de la Cruz, Robert DeMello, Navneet Dhillon, Sharmila Dissanaike, David Donson, Adolf Etchegaray, Alea Eusebio, Priscilla A. Frase, David Frenz, Kristin Gaumer, Yohannes Gebreegziabher, Anil Gehi, Tony George, L.M. Gotanco, Parul Goyal, Alex Grimm, Rajeev Gupta, Ahmad Halim, Sue Hall, David Hasselbacher, Tamra Heimert, Michelle Higley, Dan Hoit, Eric Jackson, Tim Jackson, Sundar Jayaraman, Pei-Ni Jone, Aarchan Joshi, Rajni K. Jutla, Faiyaz Kapadi, Seth Karp, Aaron S. Kesselheim, Sana Khan, Andrew Pin-wei Ko, Francis Kong, Paul Konitzky, Warren S. Krackov, Benjamin H.S. Lau, Ann LaCasce, Connie Lee, Scott Lee, Guillermo Lehmann, Kevin Leung, Paul Levett, Warren Levinson, Eric Ley, Ken Lin,

Pavel Lobanov, J. Mark Maddox, Aram Mardian, Samir Mehta, Gil Melmed, Joe Messina, Robert Mosca, Michael Murphy, Vivek Nandkarni, Siva Naraynan, Carvell Nguyen, Linh Nguyen, Deanna Nobleza, Craig Nodurft, George Noumi, Darin T. Okuda, Adam L. Palance, Paul Pamphrus, Jinha Park, Sonny Patel, Ricardo Pietrobon, Riva L. Rahl, Aashita Randeria, Rachan Reddy, Beatriu Reig, Marilou Reyes, Jeremy Richmon, Tai Roe, Rick Roller, Rajiv Roy, Diego Ruiz, Anthony Russell, Sanjay Sahgal, Urmimala Sarkar, John Schilling, Isabell Schmitt, Daren Schuhmacher, Sonal Shah, Fadi Abu Shahin, Mae Sheikh-Ali, Edie Shen, Justin Smith, John Stulak, Lillian Su, Julie Sundaram, Rita Suri, Seth Sweetser, Antonio Talayero, Merita Tan, Mark Tanaka, Eric Taylor, Jess Thompson, Indi Trehan, Raymond Turner, Okafo Uchenna, Eric Uyguanco, Richa Varma, John Wages, Alan Wang, Eunice Wang, Andy Weiss, Amy Williams, Brian Yang, Hany Zaky, Ashraf Zaman and David Zipf.

For generously contributing images to the entire *Underground Clinical Vignette* Step 2 series, we collectively thank the staff at Blackwell Science in Oxford, Boston, and Berlin as well as:

- Axford, J. *Medicine.* Osney Mead: Blackwell Science Ltd, 1996. Figures 12.28c, 12.37a, 12.37b, 12.37c, 14.20e, 14.20f, 14.46a, 14.46b, 14.47d, 14.47e, 14.47f, 14.51e, 14.58a, 14.59f, 14.6b, 14.7h, 14.7i, 14.7j, 14.7k, 14.7l, 2.103a, 2.110b, 2.110c, 2.112a, 2.112b, 2.69a, 2.90b, 2.92a, 2.92c, 2.94a, 3.20b, 3.25b, 3.35e, 6.13b, 9.9b, 9.9c, 9.9f, 12.16, 14.13, 14.15, 14.17, 14.26, 14.37, 14.44, 14.46, 14.48, 14.49, 14.55, 14.60, 14.61, 14.63, 14.65, 14.67, 14.8, 2.10c, 2.11, 2.33, 2.33b, 2.40, 2.45, 2.46, 3.13b, 3.20, 3.20c, 3.36, 3.37, 6.9.

- Bannister B, Begg N, Gillespie S. *Infectious Disease, 2nd Edition.* Osney Mead: Blackwell Science Ltd, 2000. Figures 11.3, 11.6a, 13.17, 19.6, 24.4a, 5.10a, 5.20, 5.21, 6.7, 6.8.

- Berg D. *Advanced Clinical Skills and Physical Diagnosis.* Osney Mead: Blackwell Science Inc., 1998. Figures 11, 12, 14, 15, 16, 17, 19, 39, 47, 6.

- Cuschieri A, Hennessy TPJ, Greenhalgh RM, Rowley DA, Grace PA. *Clinical Surgery.* Osney Mead: Blackwell Science Ltd, 1996. Figures 1.25, 12.1, 12.5a, 13.30, 13.35b, 13.36, 13.49, 13.50, 13.51, 15.13, 17.10, 17.21, 17.4, 17.5a, 17.5b, 22.9.

- Duckworth T. *Lecture Notes on Orthopaedics and Fractures, 3rd Edition.* Osney Mead: Blackwell Science Ltd., 2000. Figures 23.1, 23.2, 24.2, 26.1, 27.3, 29.2a, 29.2b, 40.2.

- Elliott T, Hastings M, Desselberger U. *Lecture Notes on Medical Microbiology, 3rd Edition.* Osney Mead: Blackwell Science Ltd, 1997. Figures 54, 55, 60, 63.
- Ginsberg L. *Lecture Notes on Neurology, 7th Edition.* Osney Mead: Blackwell Science Ltd, 1999. Figures 17.2, 17.5, 17.7.
- Mehta AB, Hoffbrand AV. *Haematology at a Glance.* Osney Mead: Blackwell Science Ltd, 2000. Figures 11.3, 25.2, 27.2, 29.1, 29.3, 30.2.
- Rudolf MCJ, Levene MI. *Paediatrics and Child Health.* Osney Mead: Blackwell Science Ltd, 1999. Figures 3.12, 4.1, 5.15, 5.18a, 5.51, 6.3a, 6.3b, 228b, 238.

Please let us know if your name has been missed or misspelled and we will be happy to make the update in the next edition.

PREFACE TO THE 2ND EDITION

We were very pleased with the overwhelmingly positive student feedback for the 1st edition of our *Underground Clinical Vignettes* series. Well over 100,000 copies of the UCV books are in print and have been used by students all over the world.

Over the last two years we have accumulated and incorporated **over a thousand "updates"** and improvements suggested by you, our readers, including:

- many additions of specific boards and wards testable content
- deletions of redundant and overlapping cases
- reordering and reorganization of all cases in both series
- a new master index by case name in each Atlas
- correction of a few factual errors
- diagnosis and treatment updates
- addition of 5–20 new cases in every book
- and the addition of clinical exam photographs within *UCV—Anatomy*

And most important of all, the second edition sets now include two brand new **COLOR ATLAS** supplements, one for each Clinical Vignette series.

- The *UCV–Basic Science Color Atlas* (*Step 1*) includes over 250 color plates, divided into gross pathology, microscopic pathology (histology), hematology, and microbiology (smears).
- The *UCV–Clinical Science Color Atlas* (*Step 2*) has over 125 color plates, including patient images, dermatology, and funduscopy.

Each atlas image is descriptively captioned and linked to its corresponding Step 1 case, Step 2 case, and/or Step 2 MiniCase.

For your convenience, a **Master Case Index** is located in the back of each Atlas.

How Atlas Links Work:

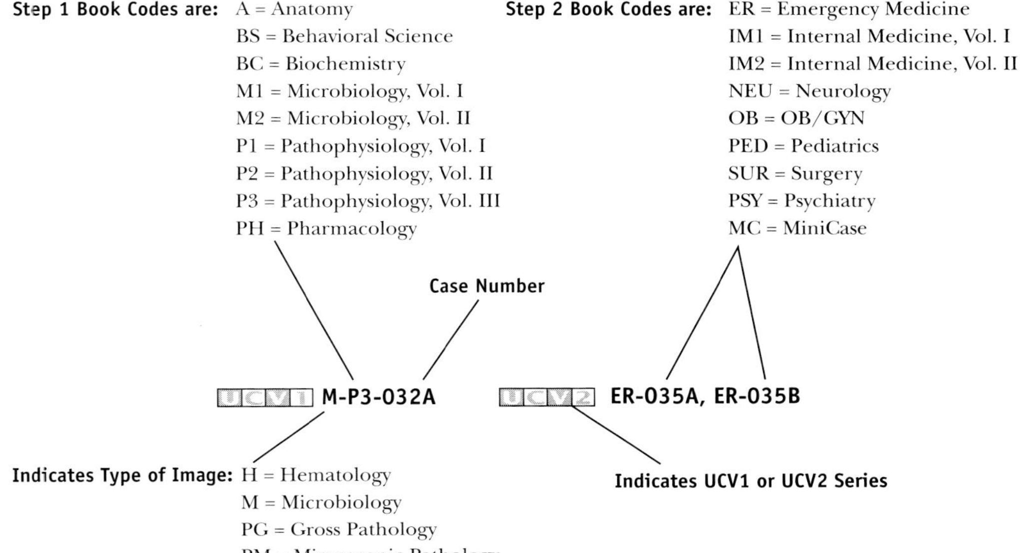

- If the Case number (032, 035, etc.) is not followed by a letter, then there is only one image. Otherwise A, B, C, D indicate up to 4 images.

Bold Faced Links: In order to give you access to the largest number of images possible, we have chosen to cross link the Step 1 and 2 series.

- If the link is bold-faced this indicates that the link is direct (i.e., Step 1 Case with the Basic Science Step 1 Atlas link).
- If the link is not bold-faced this indicates that the link is indirect (Step 1 case with Clinical Science Step 2 Atlas link or vice versa).

We have also implemented a few structural changes upon your request:

- Each current and future edition of our popular *First Aid for the USMLE Step 1* (Appleton & Lange/McGraw-Hill) and *First Aid for the USMLE Step 2* (Appleton & Lange/McGraw-Hill) book will be linked to the corresponding UCV case.
- We eliminated UCV → First Aid links as they frequently become out of date, as the *First Aid* books are revised yearly.

- The Color Atlas is also specially designed for quizzing—captions are descriptive and do not give away the case name directly.

We hope the updated UCV series will remain a unique and well-integrated study tool that provides compact clinical correlations to basic science information. They are designed to be easy and fun (comparatively) to read, and helpful for both licensing exams and the wards.

We invite your corrections and suggestions for the fourth edition of these books. For the first submission of each factual correction or new vignette that is selected for inclusion in the fourth edition, you will receive a personal acknowledgment in the revised book. If you submit over 20 high-quality corrections, additions or new vignettes we will also consider **inviting you to become a "Contributor" on the book of your choice**. If you are interested in becoming a potential "Contributor" or "Author" on a future UCV book, or working with our team in developing additional books, please also e-mail us your CV/resume.

We prefer that you submit corrections or suggestions via electronic mail to **UCVteam@yahoo.com**. Please include "Underground Vignettes" as the subject of your message. If you do not have access to e-mail, use the following mailing address: Blackwell Publishing, Attn: UCV Editors, 350 Main Street, Malden, MA 02148, USA.

Vikas Bhushan
Vishal Pall
Tao Le
October 2001

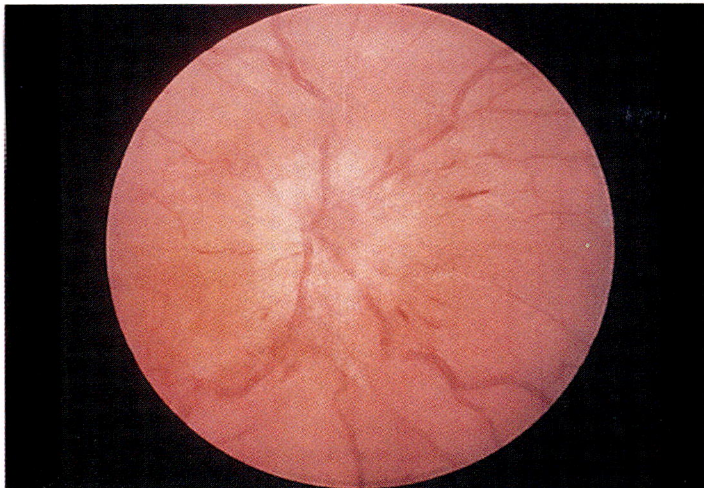

Figure ER-005
Edematous optic disk with indistinct margins, microvascular congestion, and flame hemorrhages.

Text Links:
UCV2 **ER-005**
UCV1 P1-018

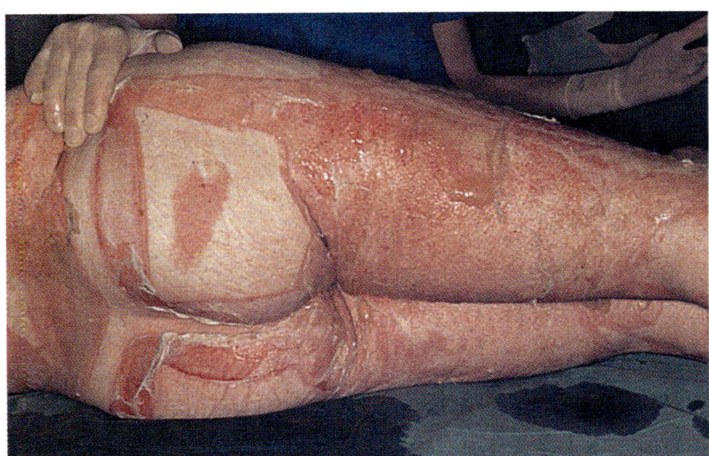

Figure ER-021A
Pink moist bullae with sloughing of the epidermis.

Text Link:
UCV2 **ER-021**

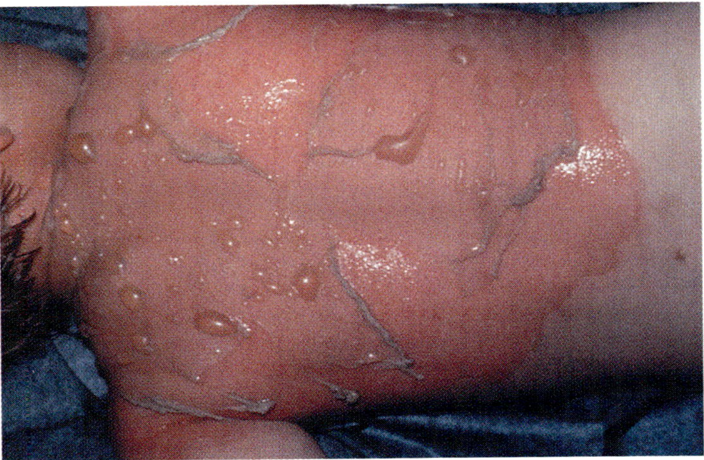

Figure ER-021B
Well-demarcated pink, moist bullae with large erosions and sloughing of the epidermis.

Text Link:
UCV2 **ER-021**

Figure ER-021C
Incision lines through a full-thickness burn.

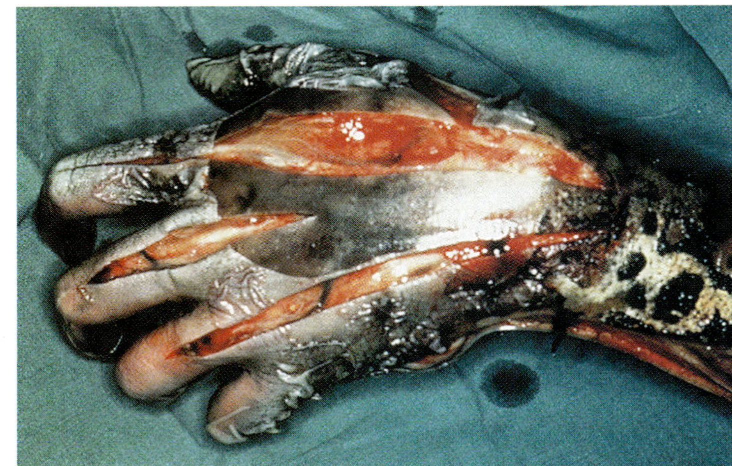

Text Link:
UCV2 **ER-021**

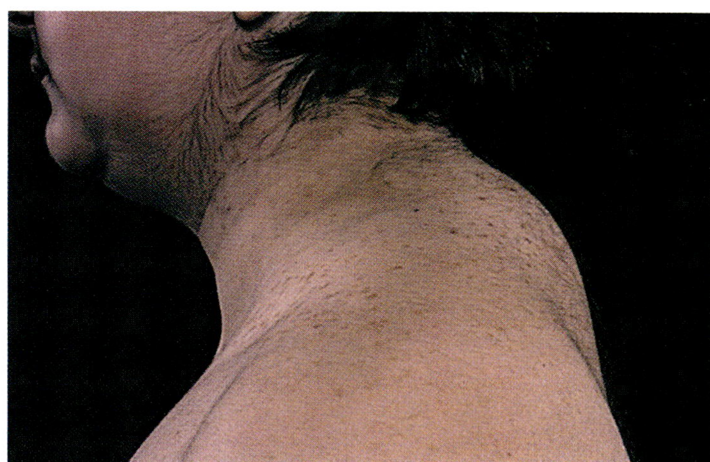

Figure IM1-019A
Large soft tissue mass overlying the interscapular area (buffalo hump).

Text Links:
UCV2 **IM1-019**
UCV1 P1-049

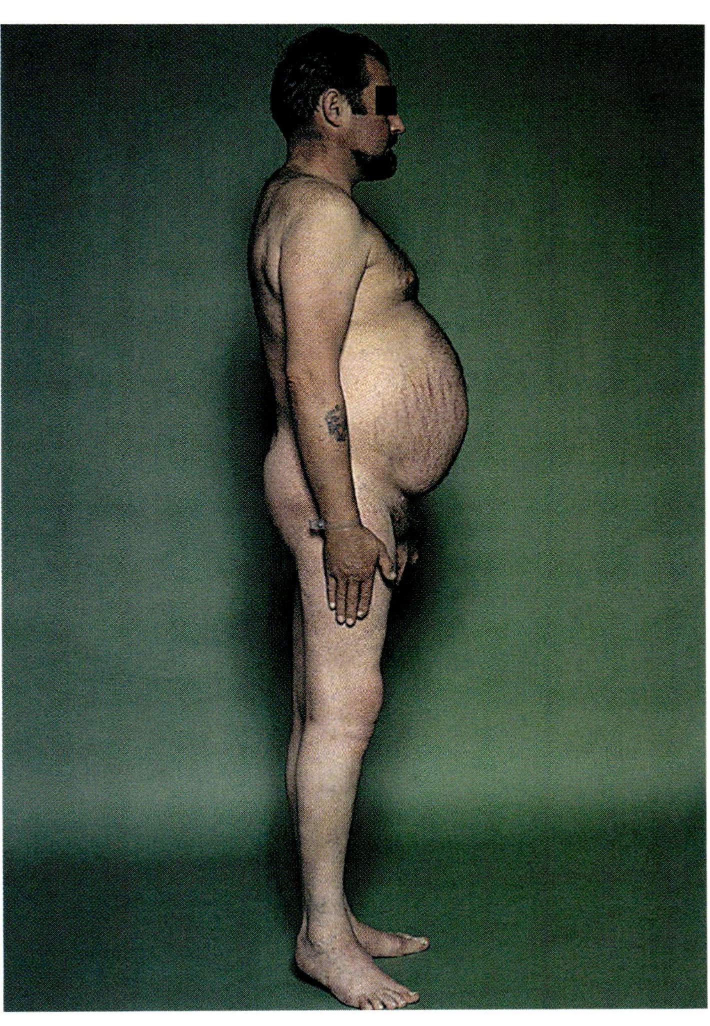

Figure IM1-019B
Truncal obesity with peripheral wasting ("lemon-on-stick" appearance).

Text Links:
UCV2 **IM1-019**
UCV1 P1-049

Figure IM1-019C
Truncal obesity with purple vertical striae along the abdomen.

Text Links:
UCV2 **IM1-019**
UCV1 P1-049

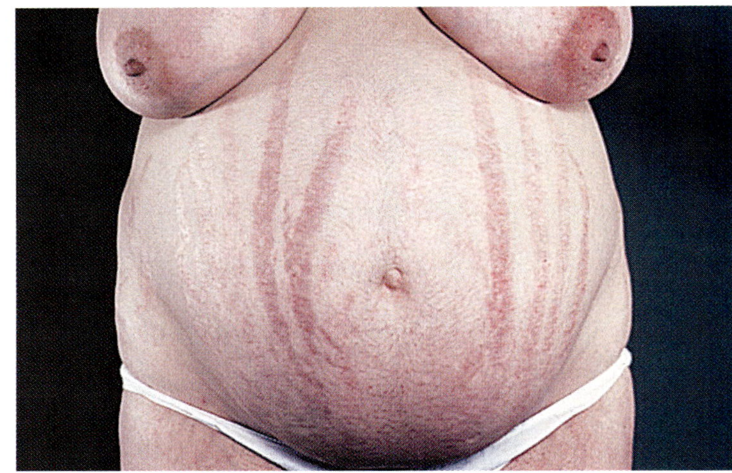

Figure IM1-019D
Moon-shaped plethoric facies.

Text Links:
UCV2 **IM1-019**
UCV1 P1-049

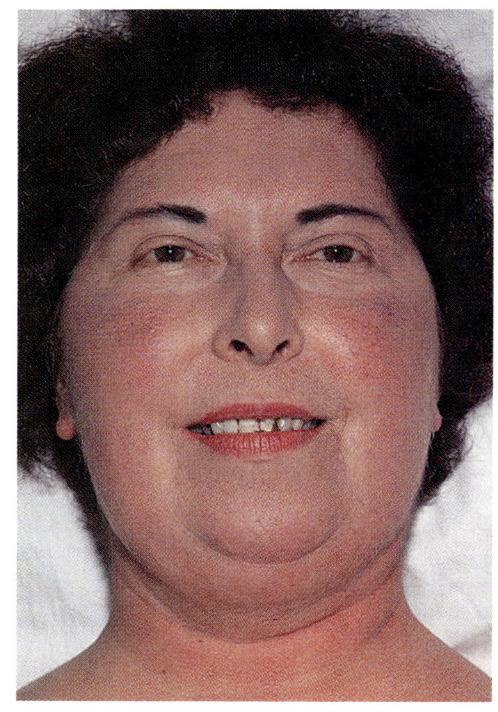

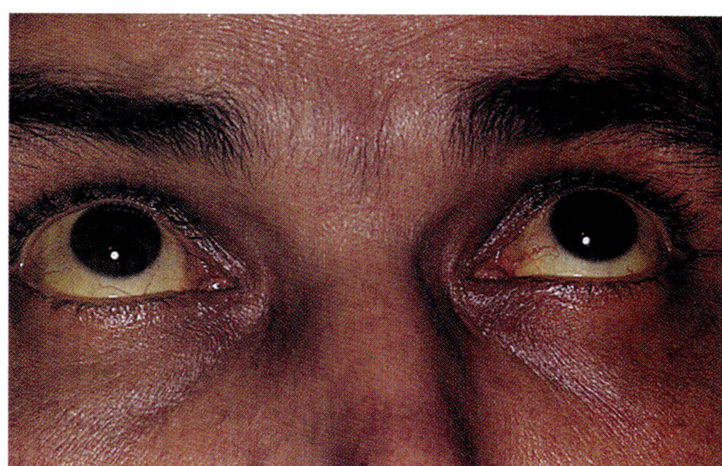

Figure IM1-034A
Yellow sclera (icterus).

Text Links:
UCV2 **IM1-034**
UCV1 P1-091

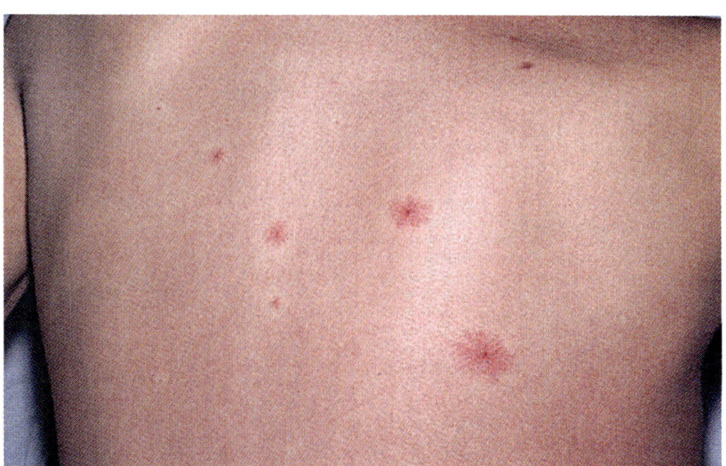

Figure IM1-034B
Multiple central dilated arterioles with radiating blood vessels (spider angiomata).

Text Links:
UCV2 **IM1-034**
UCV1 P1-091

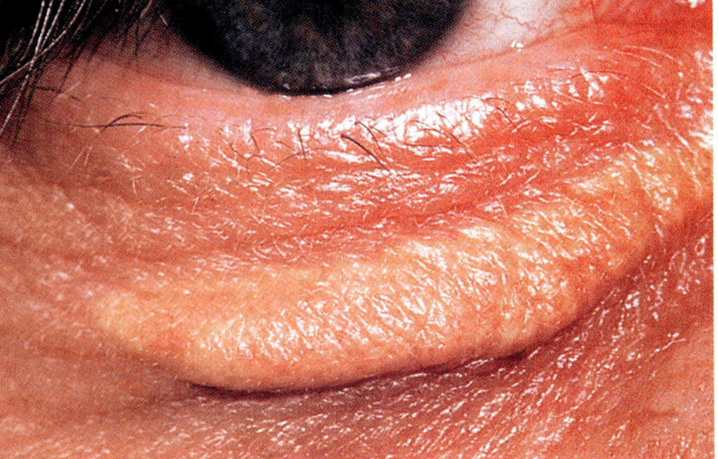

Figure IM1-039
Soft yellow infra-orbital plaque (xanthelasma).

Text Links:
UCV2 **IM1-039**
UCV1 P1-100

Figure IM1-043
Atrophic, bald, beefy-red tongue.

Text Links:
UCV2 **IM1-043**
UCV1 BC-077

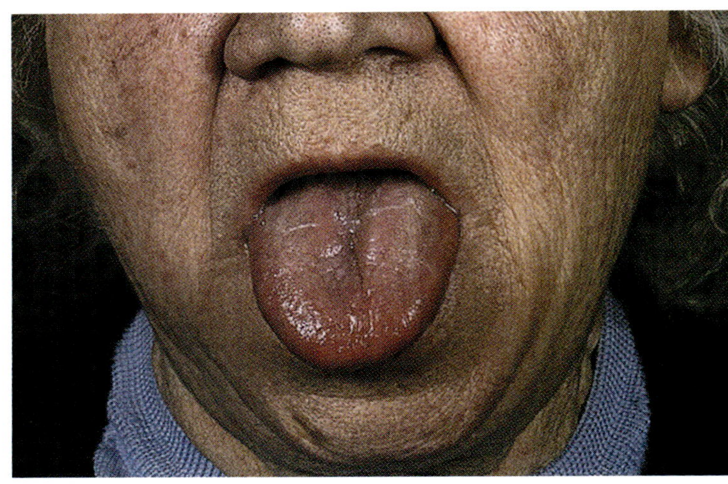

Figure IM1-052
Dusky cyanosis and erythematous facies.

Text Links:
UCV2 **IM1-052**
UCV1 P2-034

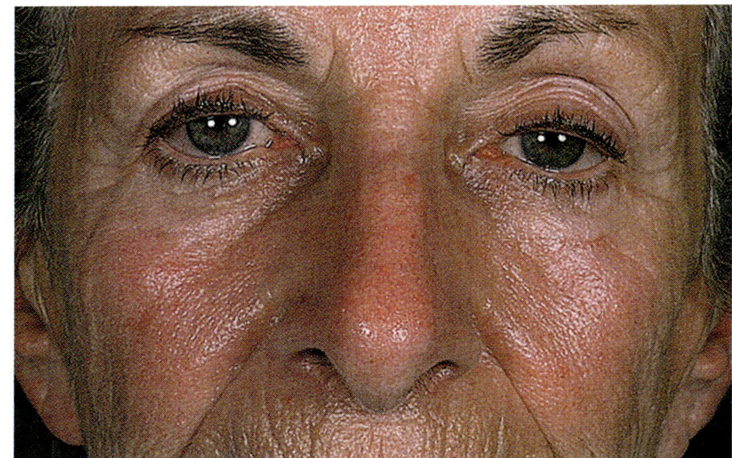

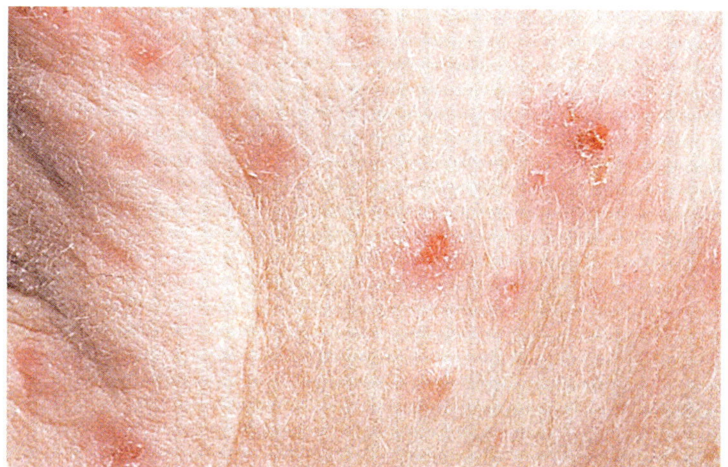

Figure IM2-005
Intensely pruritic, excoriations (ruptured vesiculo-pustular lesions) atop erythematous base.

Text Links:
UCV2 **IM2-005**
UCV1 P1-033

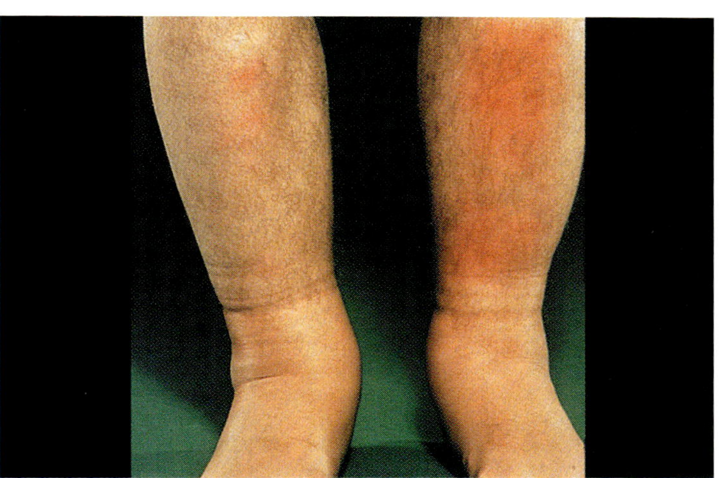

Figure IM2-006
Multiple, tender erythematous plaques and nodules on the shins.

Text Link:
UCV2 **IM2-006**

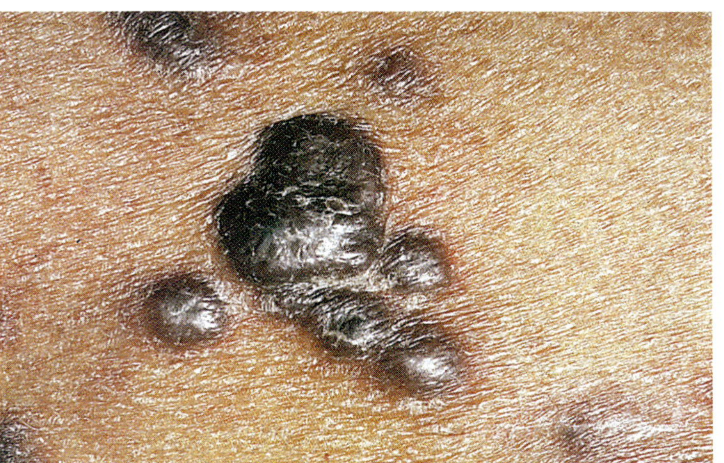

Figure IM2-007
Raised dusky, purple nodules and papules.

Text Links:
UCV2 **IM2-007**
UCV1 P1-037

Figure IM2-008A
Well demarcated plaques with silver scales.

Text Links:
UCV2 **IM2-008**
UCV1 P1-045

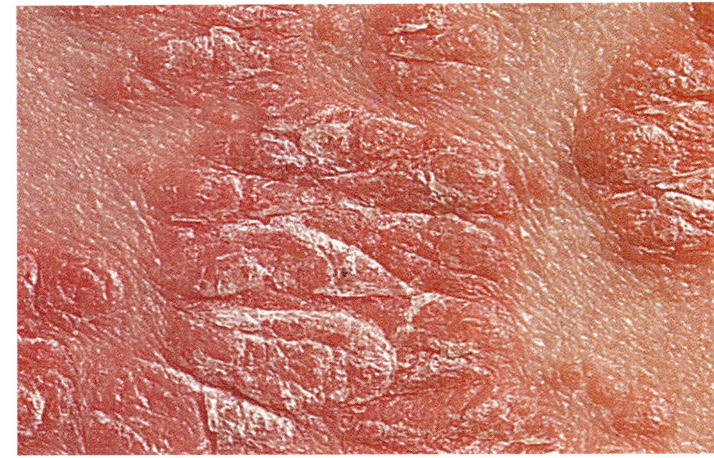

Figure IM2-008B
Pitting of nails and separation of nail plate (onycholysis).

Text Links:
UCV2 **IM2-008**
UCV1 P1-045

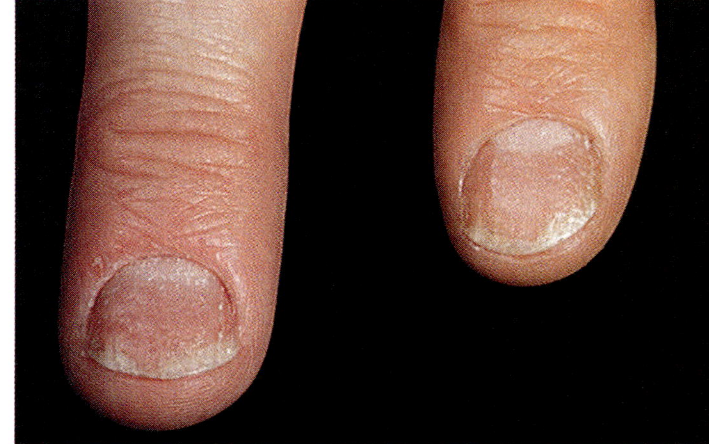

Figure IM2-008C
Erythematous plaques on the dorsum of the hand and arthropathy of the distal interphalangeal joints.

Text Links:
UCV2 **IM2-008C**
UCV1 P1-045D

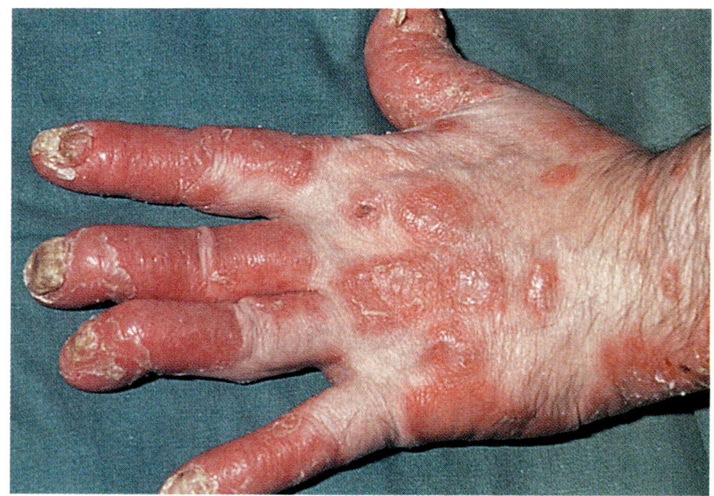

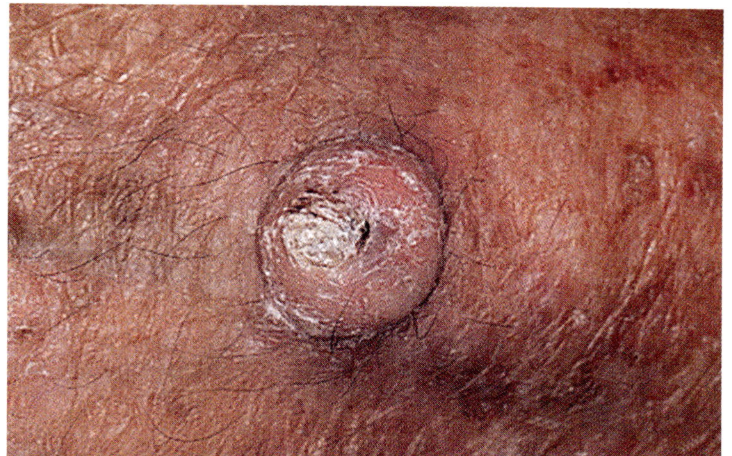

Figure IM2-010A
Skin-colored nodule with ulceration and crusting.

Text Links:
UCV2 **IM2-010**
UCV1 A-009

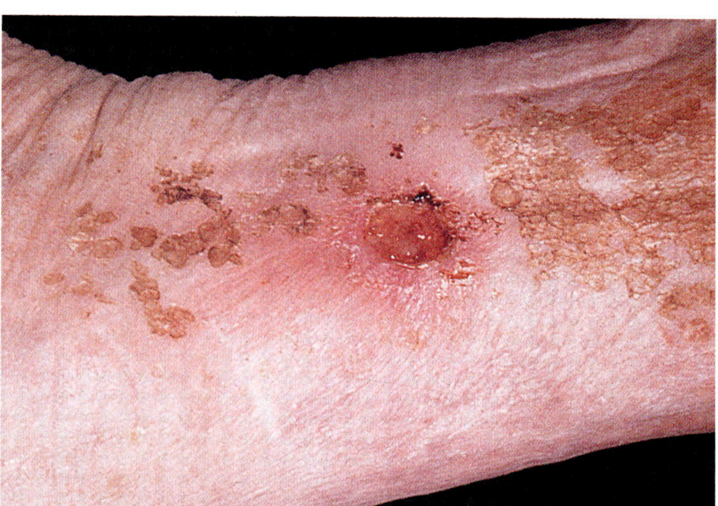

Figure IM2-010B
Sharply demarcated ulcer surrounded by changes of stasis dermatitis.

Text Links:
UCV2 **IM2-010**
UCV1 A-009

Figure IM2-011
Tall, thin male with pectus excavatum and arachnodactyly (marfanoid habitus).

Text Links:
UCV2 **IM2-011**
UCV1 P2-012

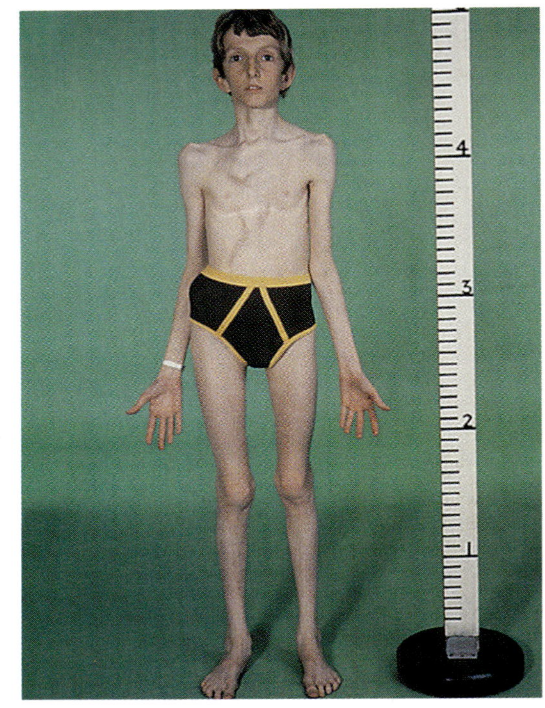

Figure IM2-018
Purulent urethral discharge.

Text Links:
UCV2 **IM2-018**
UCV1 M1-091

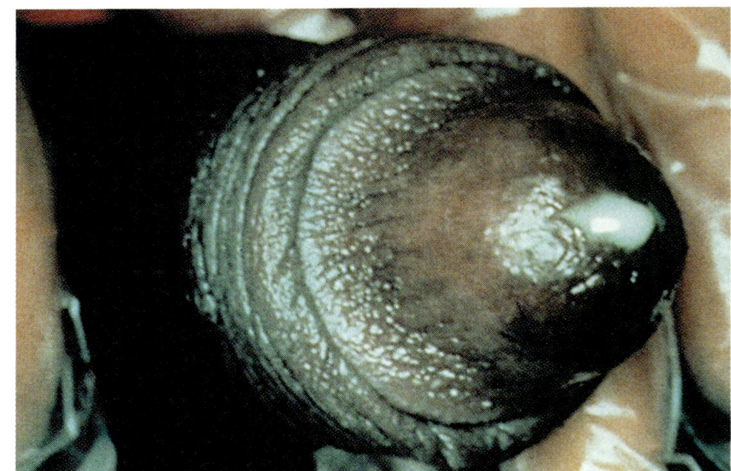

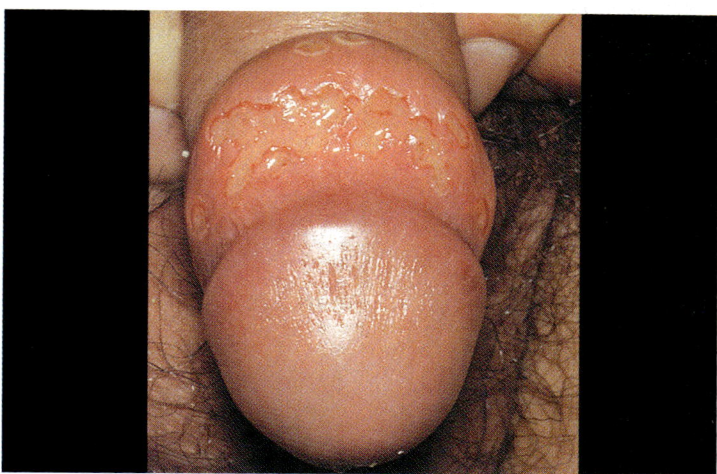

Figure IM2-019A
Vesicles coalescing to form bullae on underside of foreskin.

Text Links:
UCV2 **IM2-019**
UCV1 M1-100

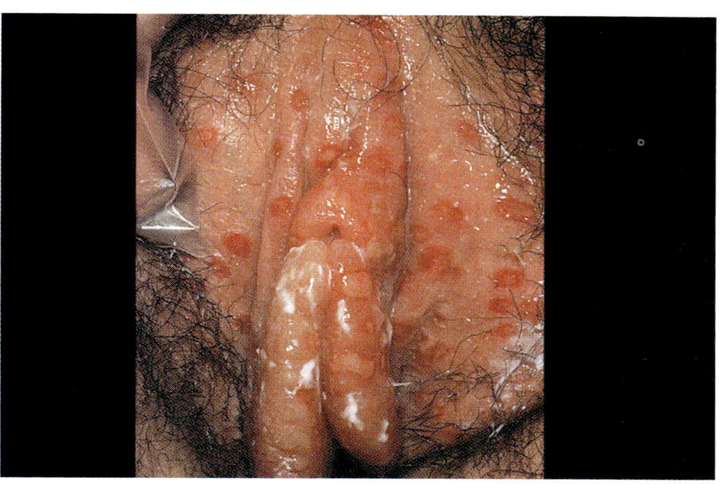

Figure IM2-019B
Multiple vesicles and erosions on the vulva.

Text Links:
UCV2 **IM2-019**
UCV1 M1-100

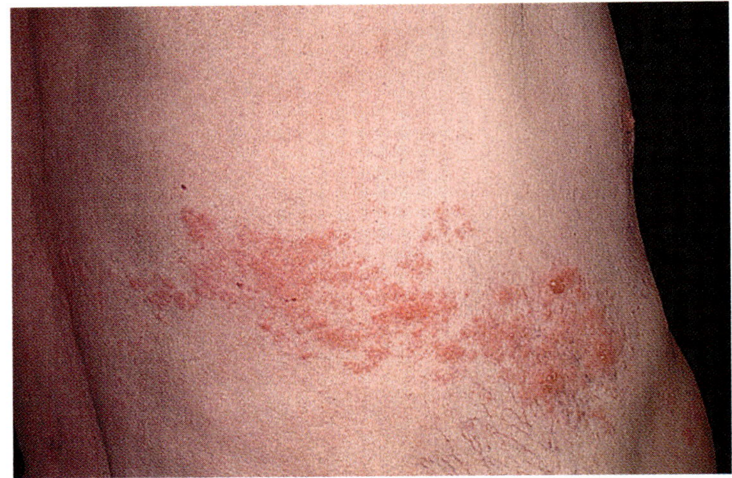

Figure IM2-020A
Painful, grouped vesicles in a unilateral dermatomal distribution.

Text Links:
UCV2 **IM2-020**
UCV1 M1-101

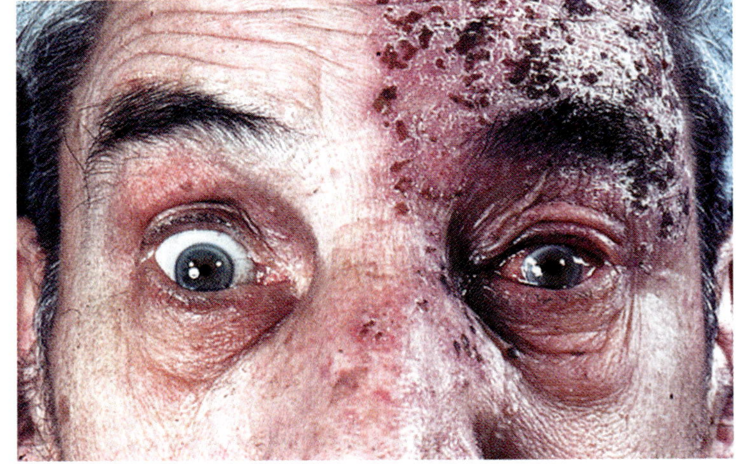

Figure IM2-020B
Crusting, ruptured vesicles and erythema in the distribution of the ophthalmic branch of the left trigeminal nerve.

Text Links:
UCV2 **IM2-020**
UCV1 M1-101

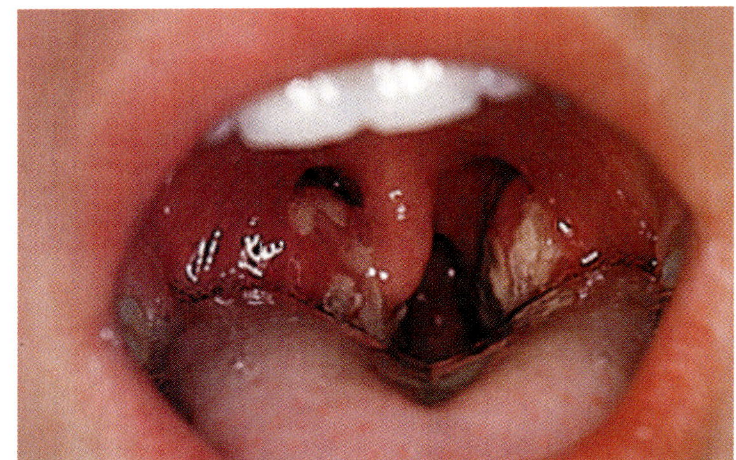

Figure IM2-022
Enlarged, erythematous tonsils with purulent exudate and uvular deviation.

Text Links:
UCV2 **IM2-022**
UCV1 M2-010

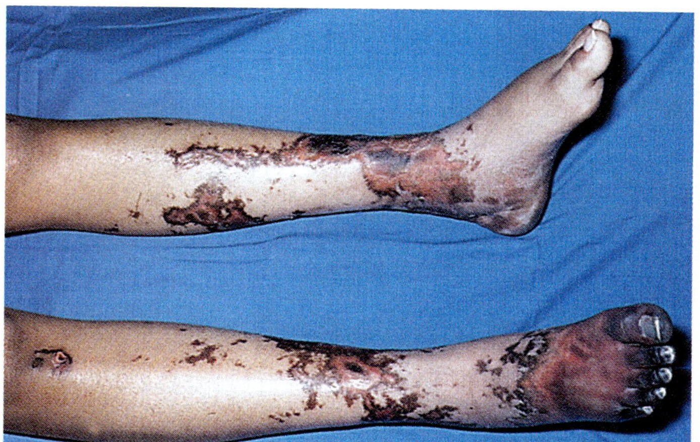

Figure IM2-024
Bilateral lower extremity purpura and necrosis of digits of the right foot.

Text Links:
UCV2 **IM2-024**
UCV1 M2-024

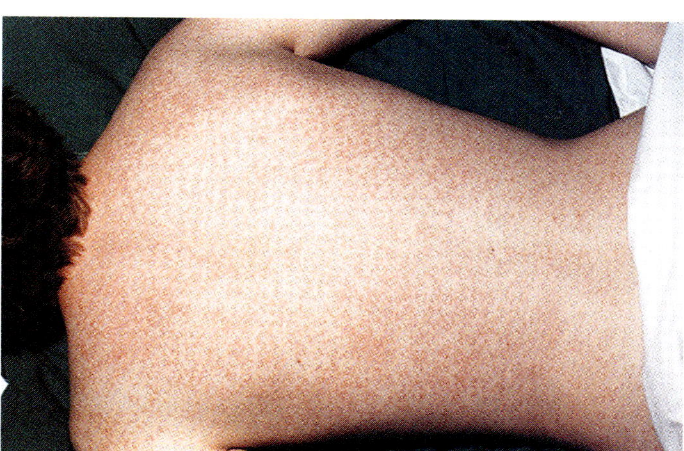

Figure IM2-026
Top to bottom spread of discrete pink macules on the trunk.

Text Links:
UCV2 **IM2-026**
UCV1 M2-047

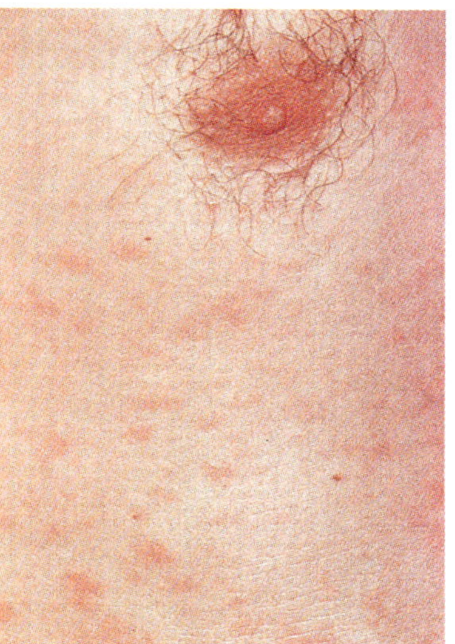

Figure IM2-027A
Diffuse macular rash on the trunk.

Text Links:
UCV2 **IM2-027**
UCV1 M2-060

Figure IM2-027B
Copper-colored macular rash on the sole.

Text Links:
UCV2 **IM2-027**
UCV1 M2-060

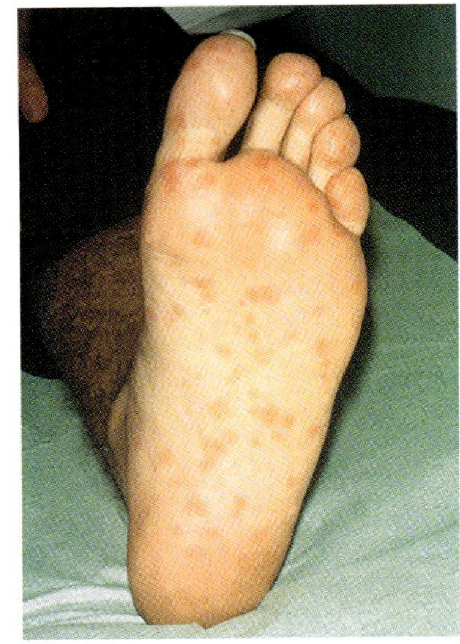

Figure IM2-028
Destruction of the right ankle joint (Charcot's joint) and foot edema.

Text Links:
UCV2 **IM2-028**
UCV1 M2-061

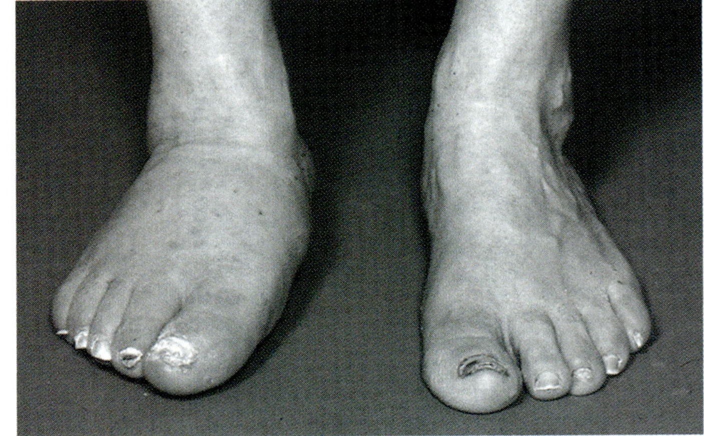

Figure IM2-030
Erythematous macules on the trunk (rose spots).

Text Links:
UCV2 **IM2-030**
UCV1 M2-070

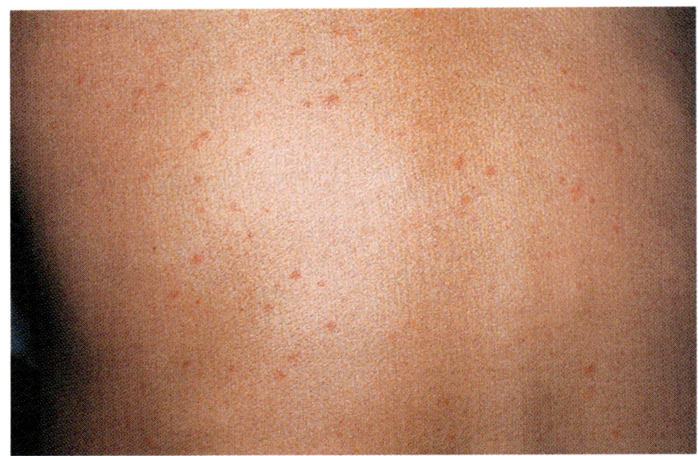

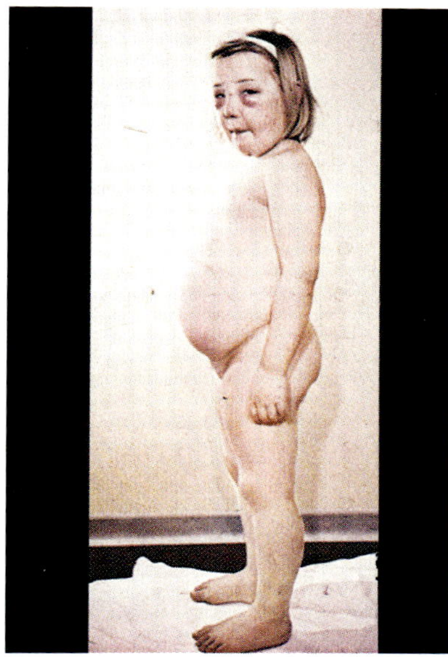

Figure IM2-036
Periorbital edema, abdominal distention, and bilateral lower extremity edema (anasarca).

Text Links:
UCV2 **IM2-036**
UCV1 P2-062

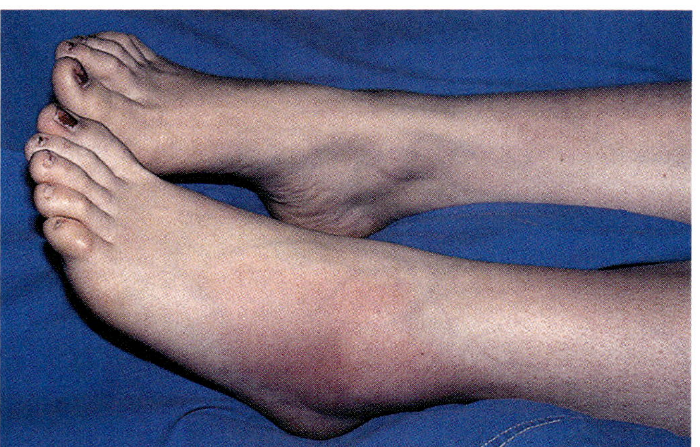

Figure IM2-041A
Edema and erythema of the left ankle.

Text Links:
UCV2 **IM2-041**
UCV1 P3-076

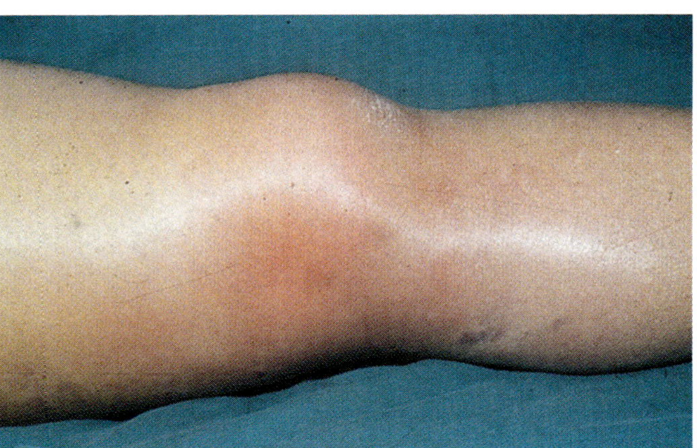

Figure IM2-041B
Unilateral swelling and erythema of the knee.

Text Links:
UCV2 **IM2-041**
UCV1 P3-076

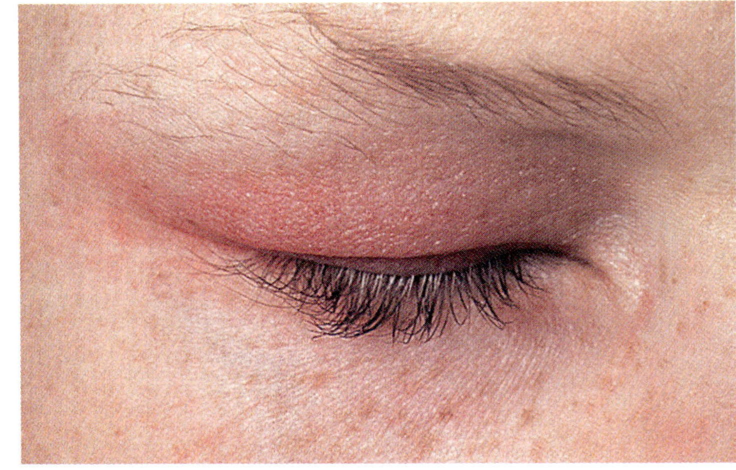

Figure IM2-051A
Violaceous discoloration and edema of the eyelid (heliotrope rash).

Text Links:
UCV2 **IM2-051**
UCV1 P3-081

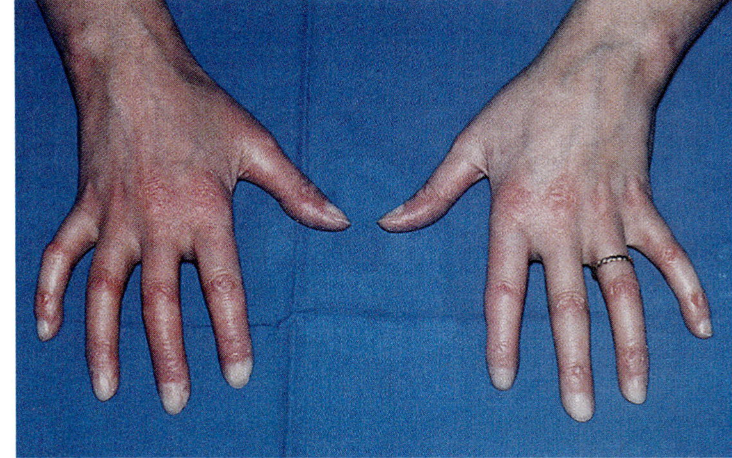

Figure IM2-051B
Bilateral, firm, erythematous papules over the extensor surfaces of the metacarpophalangeal and interphalangeal joints.

Text Links:
UCV2 **IM2-051**
UCV1 P3-081

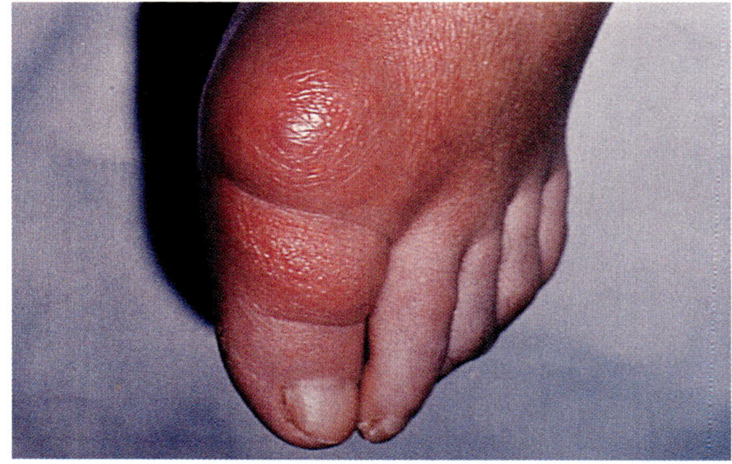

Figure IM2-052A
Erythema and swelling of the great toe (podagra).

Text Links:
UCV2 **IM2-052**
UCV1 BC-094

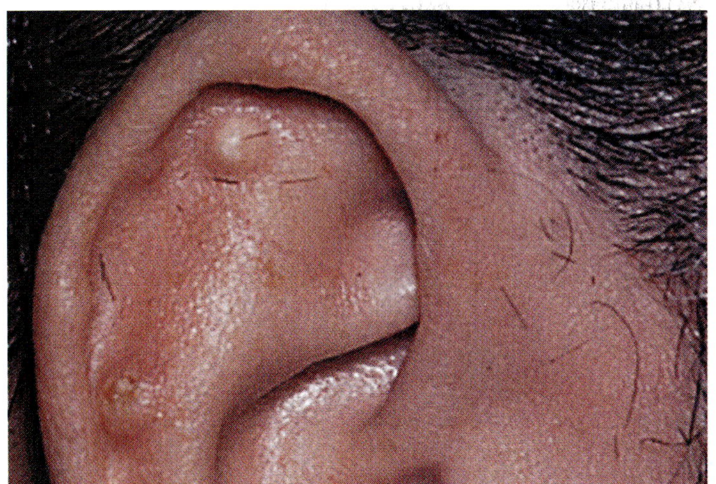

Figure IM2-052B
Yellowish-white nodules on the right ear (tophi).

Text Links:
UCV2 **IM2-052**
UCV1 BC-094

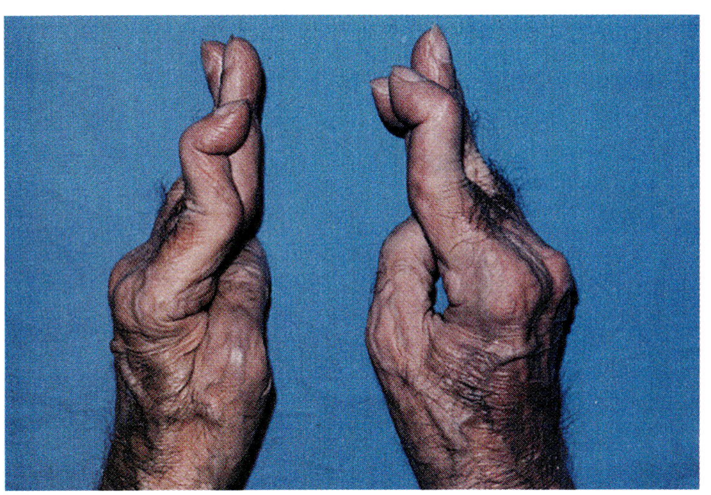

Figure IM2-055
Hyperextension of the proximal interphalangeal joints and flexion of the distal interphalangeal joints (swan neck deformity).

Text Links:
UCV2 **IM2-055**
UCV1 P3-093

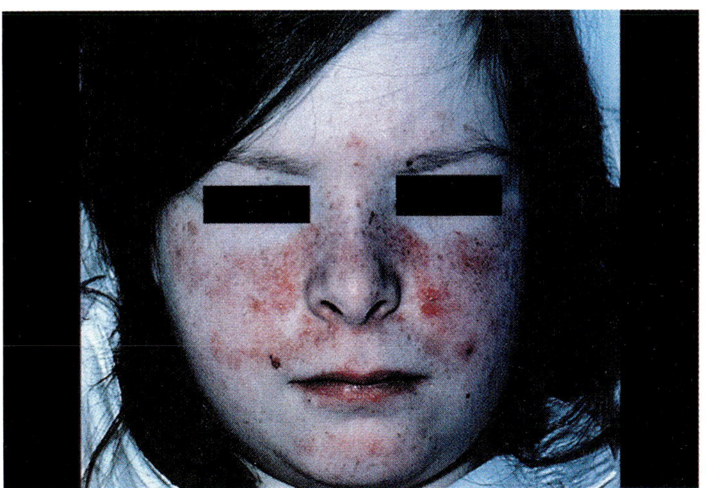

Figure IM2-056
Bilateral cheek erythema in a distribution (photosensitive malar rash).

Text Links:
UCV2 **IM2-056**
UCV1 P3-095

Figure NEU-005
Left-sided hemiplegia with flexion of the upper and lower extremities.

Text Link:
UCV2 **NEU-005**

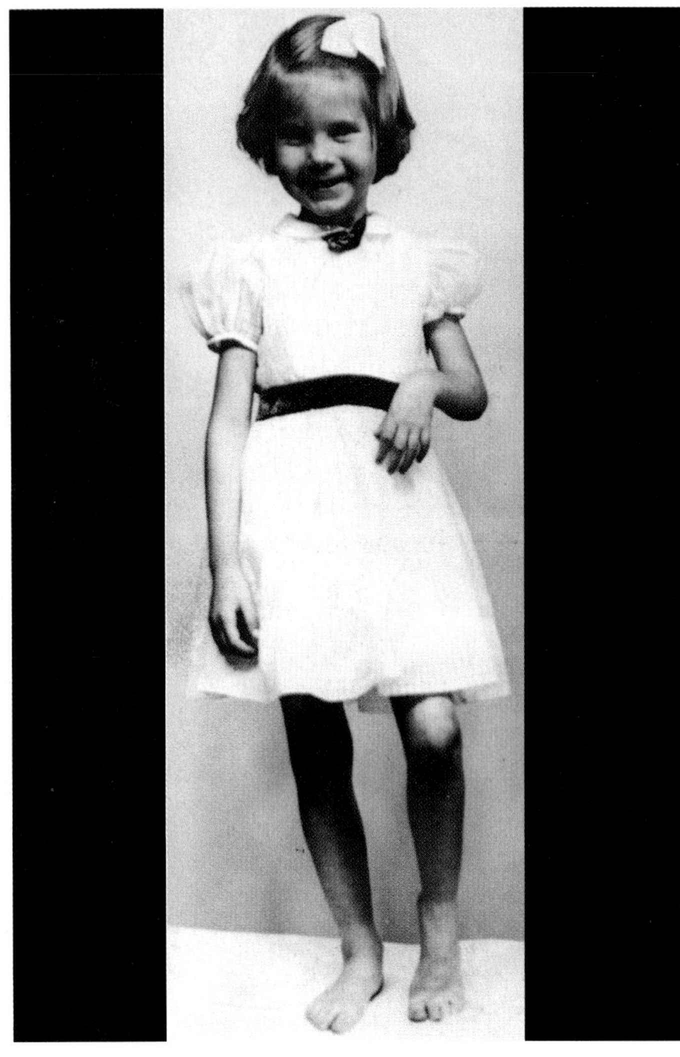

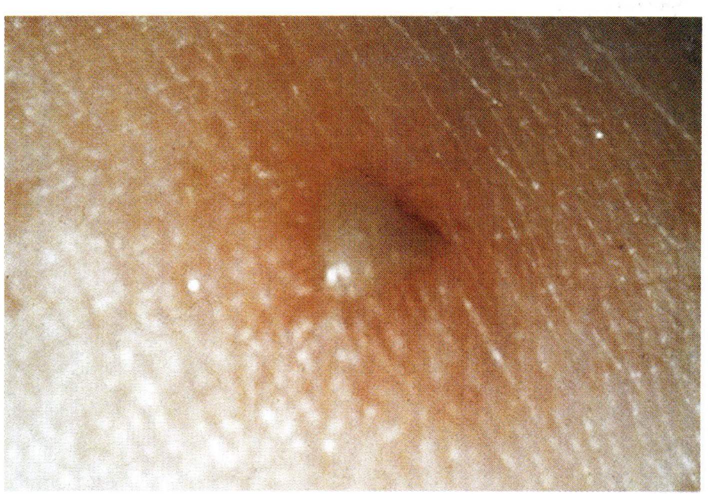

Figure OB-007
Tense vesicle with an erythematous base.

Text Link:
UCV2 **OB-007**

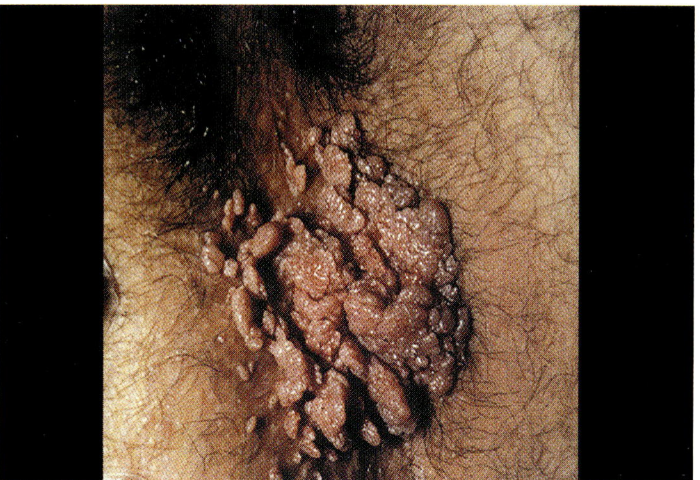

Figure OB-011A
Papillomatous perianal cauliflower-like lesions (condyloma acuminatum).

Text Links:
UCV2 **OB-011A**
UCV1 M2-103A

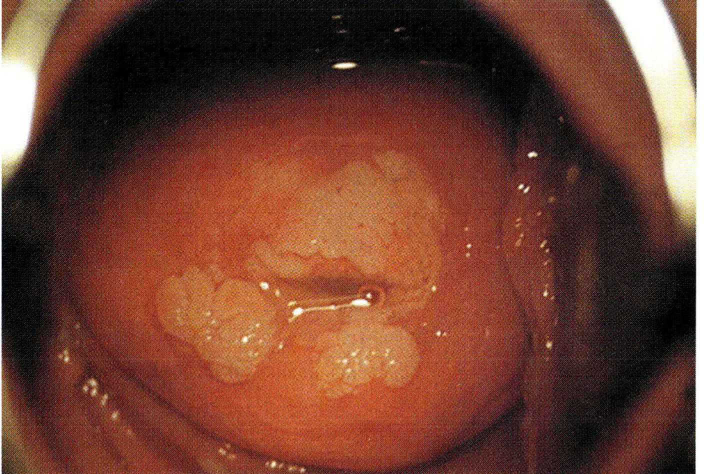

Figure OB-011B
Yellow, flat-topped cauliflower-like lesions on the cervix.

Text Links:
UCV2 **OB-011**
UCV1 M2-103

Figure OB-027A
Lower extremity petechiae.

Text Links:
UCV2 **OB-027**
UCV1 M2-106

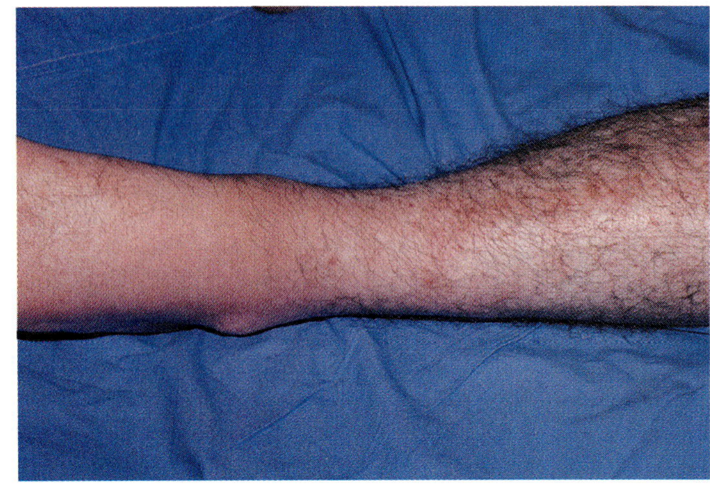

Figure OB-027B
Desquamation of hands and feet.

Text Links:
UCV2 **OB-027**
UCV1 M2-106

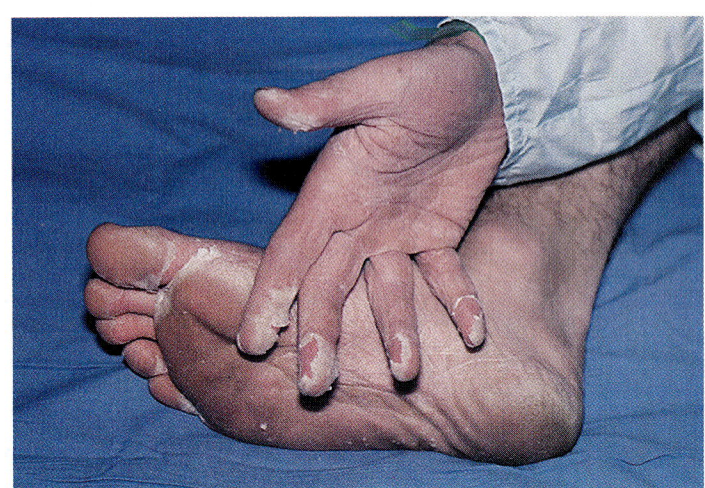

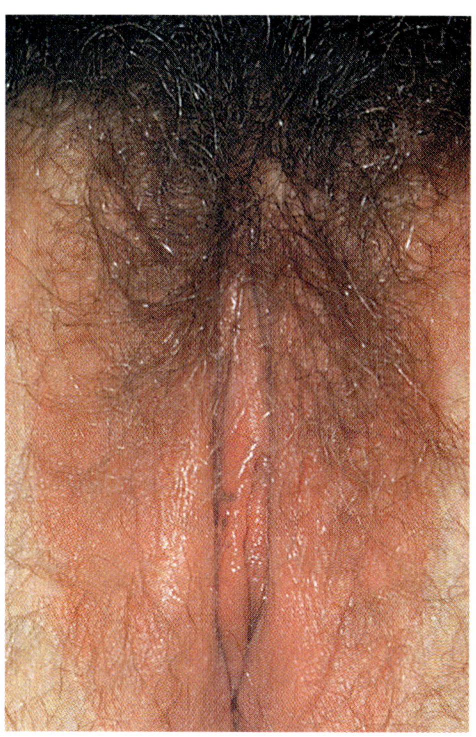

Figure OB-030
Inflammation of the vulva.

Text Link:
UCV2 **OB-030**

Figure PED-018
Swelling due to subcutaneous extravasation of blood.

Text Links:
UCV2 **PED-018**
UCV1 BC-079

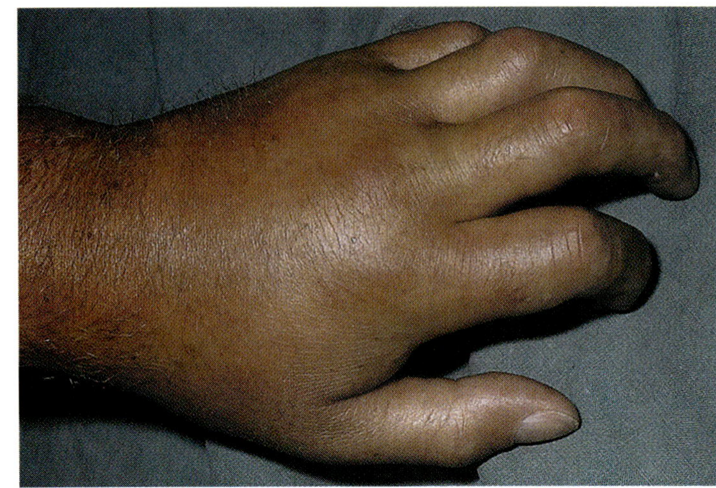

Figure PED-019A
Palpable purpura on the upper extremities, buttocks, and thighs.

Text Links:
UCV2 **PED-019**
UCV1 P2-025

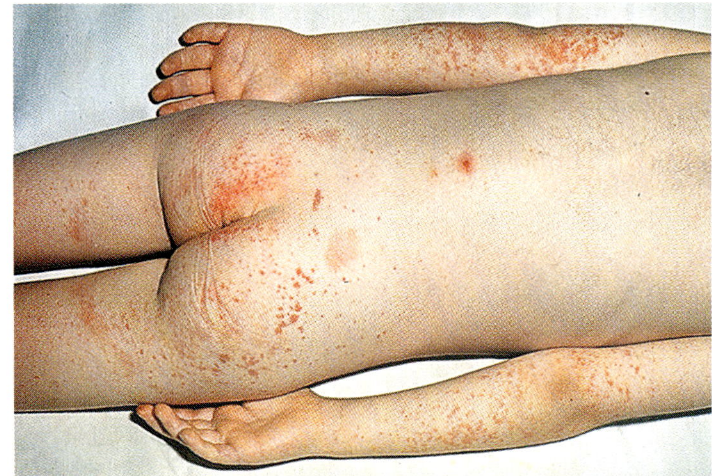

Figure PED-019B
Palpable purpura on proximal lower extremities.

Text Links:
UCV2 **PED-019**
UCV1 P2-025

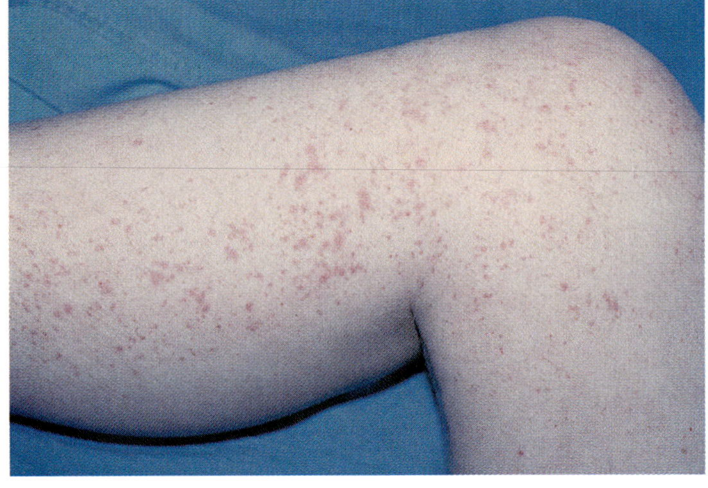

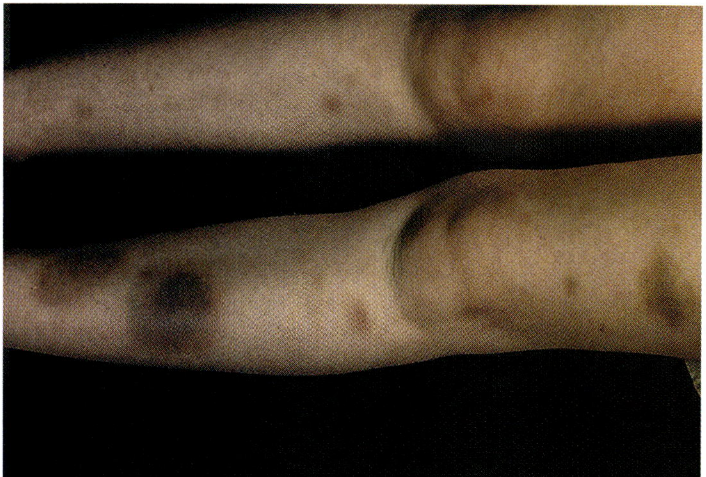

Figure PED-020: Ecchymoses of the lower extremities.

Text Links:
UCV2 **PED-020**
UCV1 P2-030

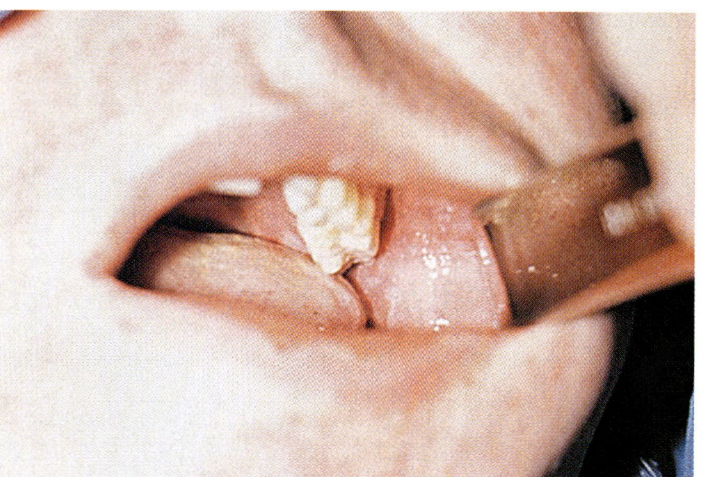

Figure PED-030A Erythematous macules with central white spots on the buccal mucosa (Koplik spots).

Text Links:
UCV2 **PED-030**
UCV1 M2-023

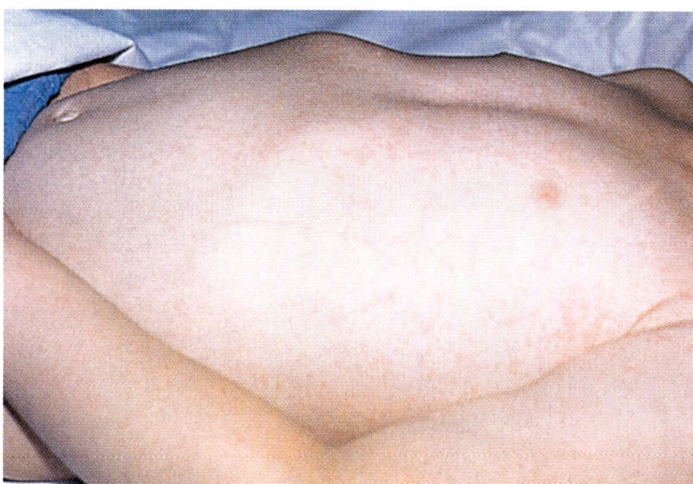

Figure PED-030B Top to bottom spread of morbilliform rash.

Text Links:
UCV2 **PED-030**
UCV1 M2-023

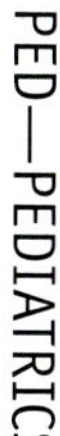

Figure PED-035
Crops of vesicles on an erythematous base (dew drops on a rose petal).

Text Links:
UCV2 **PED-035**
UCV1 M2-074

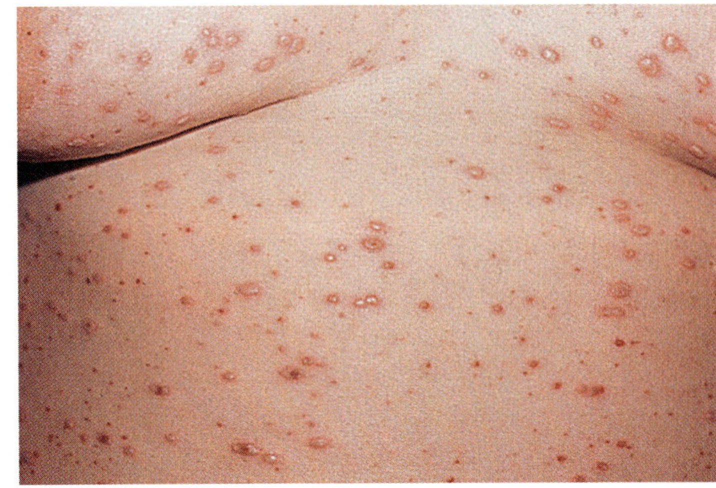

Figure PED-049
Apparent bilateral calf hypertrophy.

Text Links:
UCV2 **PED-049**
UCV1 BC-086

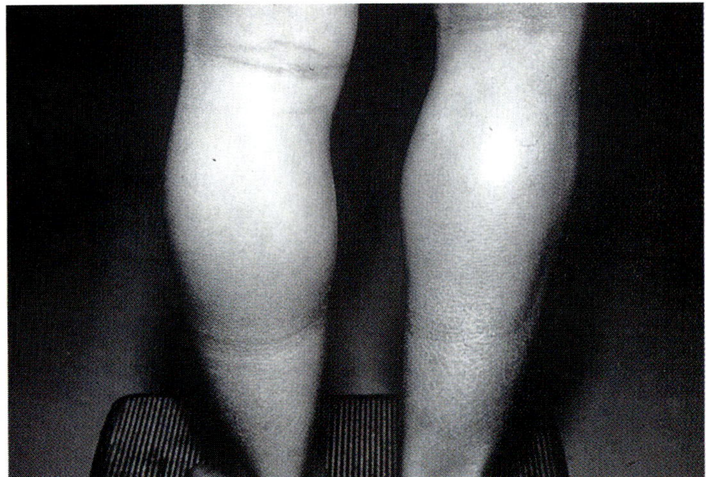

Figure PED-051A
Gradual abduction of the patient's hips as the femoral head is held between the examiner's fingers and thumb.

Text Links:
UCV2 **PED-051**
UCV1 A-086

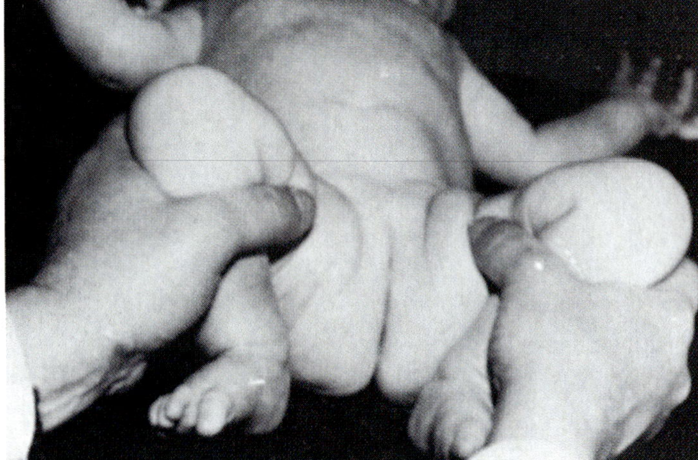

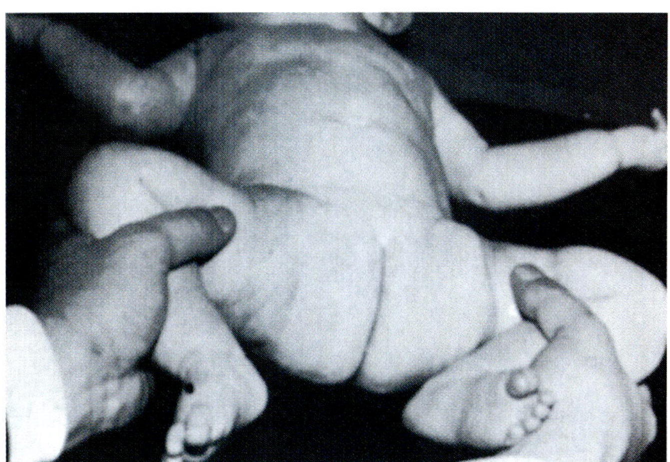

Figure PED-051B
Normal range of motion for neonatal hip abduction.

Text Links:
UCV2 **PED-051**
UCV1 A-086

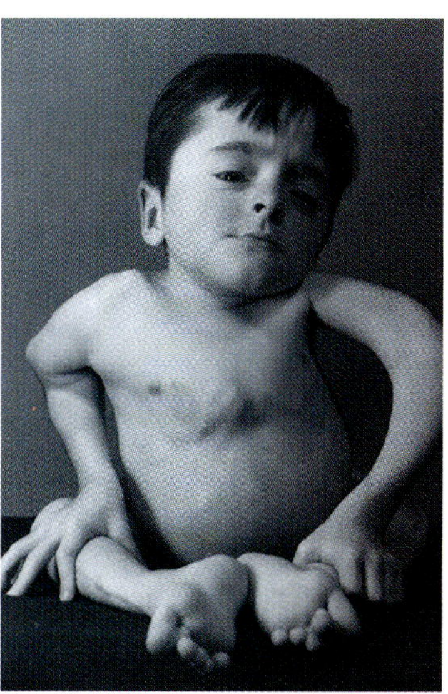

Figure PED-052
Bony deformities secondary to multiple fractures following minor trauma.

Text Links:
UCV2 **PED-052**
UCV1 BC-090

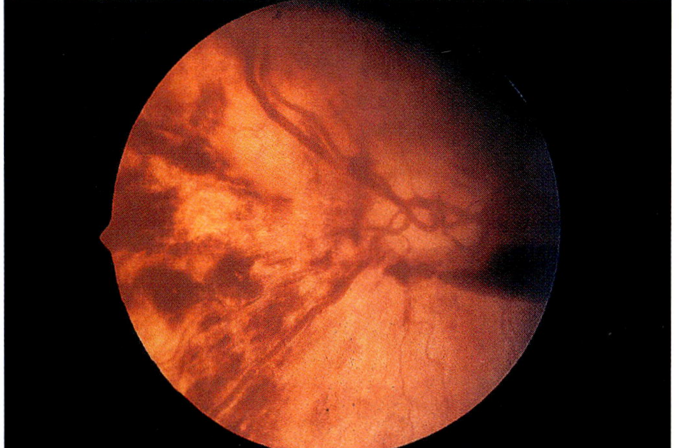

Figure PED-053
Diffuse microvascular hemorrhages.

Text Links:
UCV2 **PED-053**
UCV1 BS-034

Figure SUR-004
Irregularly pigmented macule and scaly black nodule on the sole.

Text Links:
UCV2 **PED-004**
UCV1 P1-040A

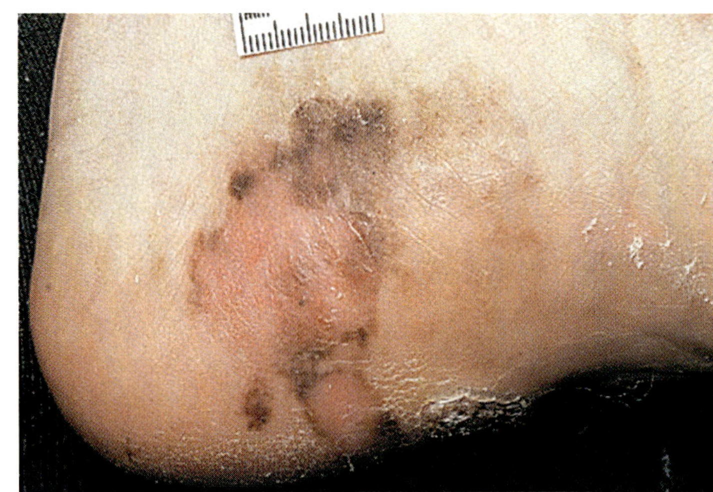

Figure SUR-018
Longitudinal tear in the mucosa of the anal canal.

Text Link:
UCV2 **SUR-018**

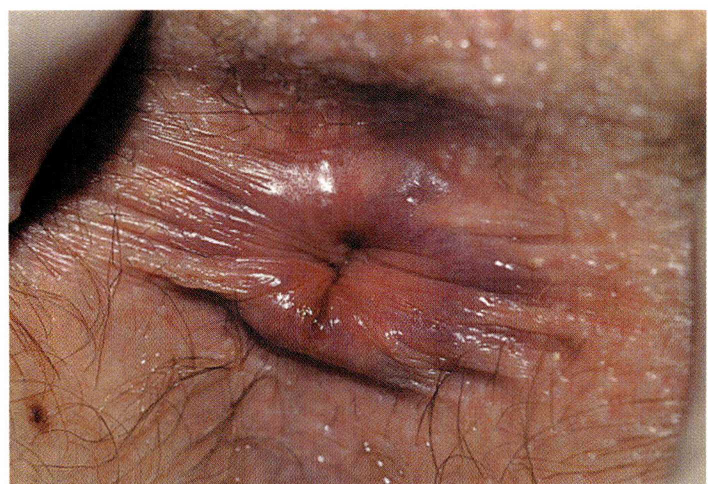

Figure SUR-021
Pedunculated mass arising from the rectal mucosa.

Text Link:
UCV2 **SUR-021**

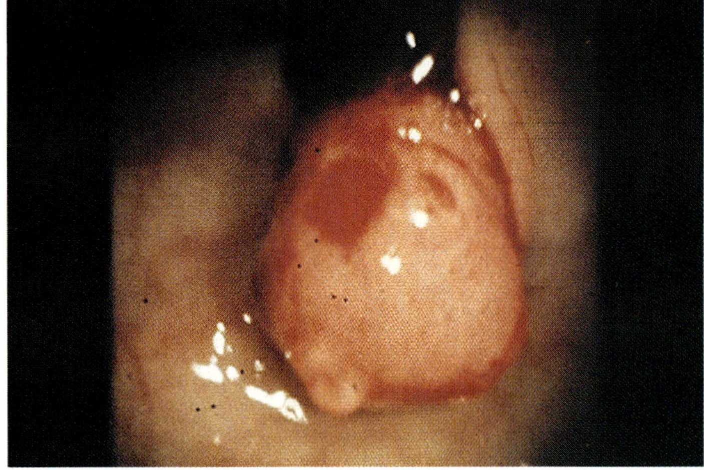

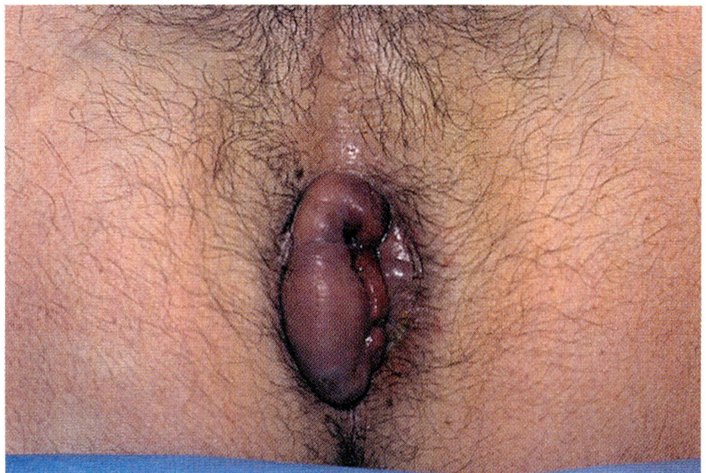

Figure SUR-028
Irreducible purplish-red nodular mass protruding from the anal canal.

Text Links:
UCV2 **SUR-028**
UCV1 A-029

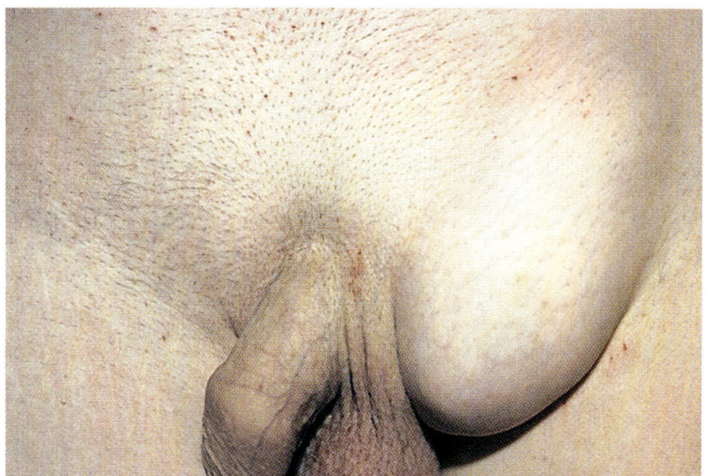

Figure SUR-029
Reducible inguinal mass protruding superiorly and medially to the pubic tubercle.

Text Links:
UCV2 **SUR-029**
UCV1 A-030

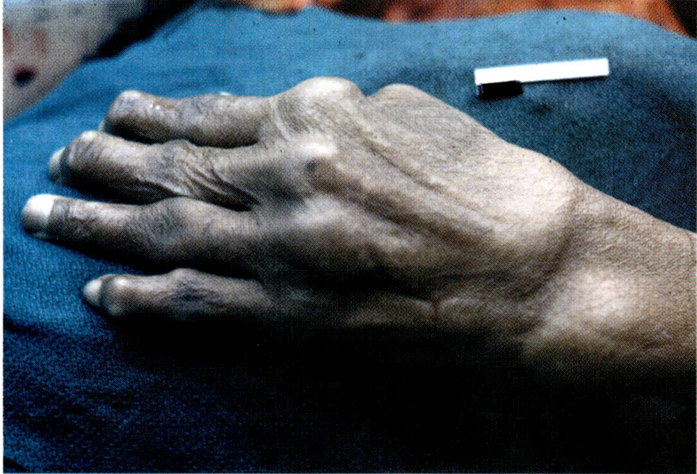

Figure SUR-044
Deforming arthritis of the carpal and interphalangeal joints with visible swellings over the distal interphalangeal joints (Heberden's nodes).

Text Links:
UCV2 **SUR-044**
UCV1 P3-073

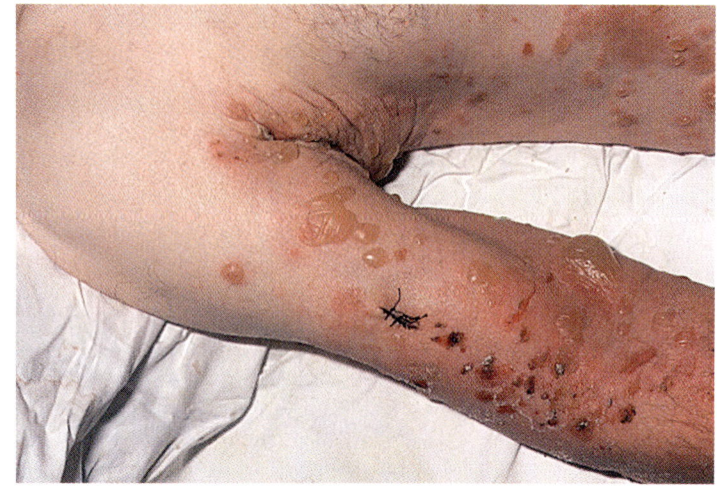

Figure MC-017
Tense bullae on erythematous base.

Text Link:
UCV2 **MC-017**

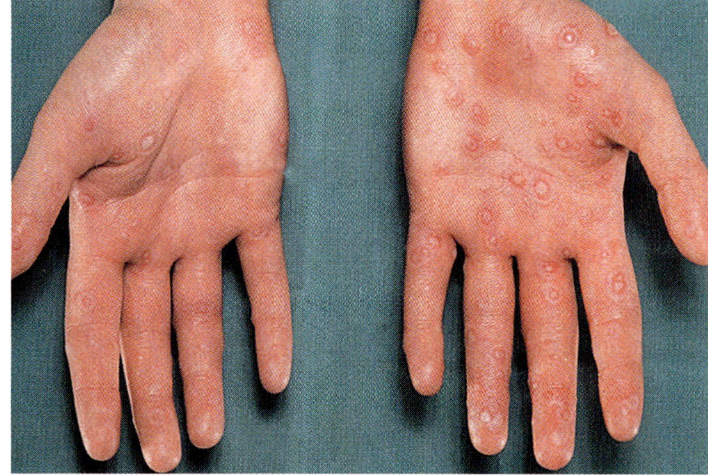

Figure MC-018
Multiple erythematous targetoid lesions on the palms.

Text Links:
UCV2 **MC-018**
UCV1 P1-035

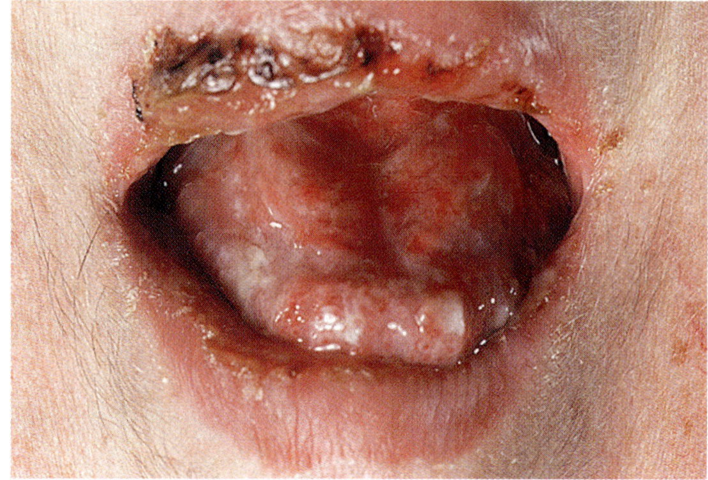

Figure MC-019
Ruptured bullae on the oral mucosa with crusting.

Text Links:
UCV2 **MC-019**
UCV1 P1-043

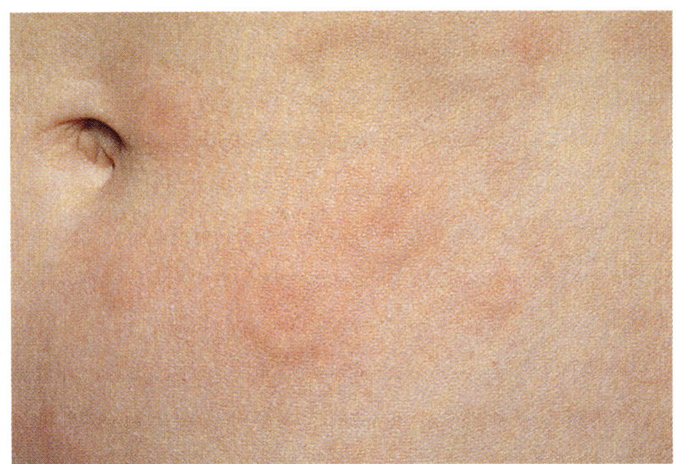

Figure MC-021
Multiple erythematous wheals with dermal edema.

Text Links:
UCV2 **MC-021**
UCV1 M1-016

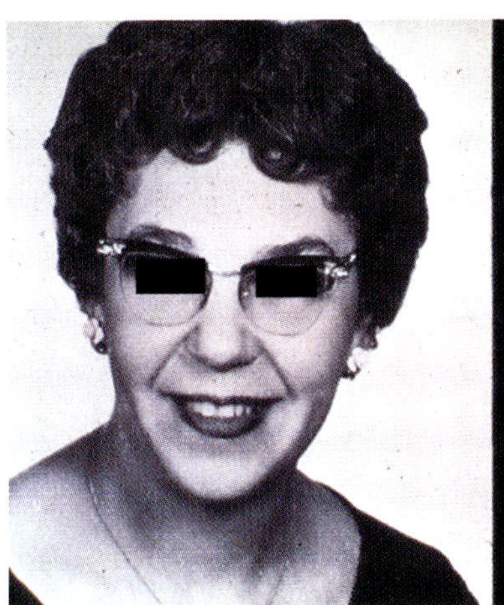
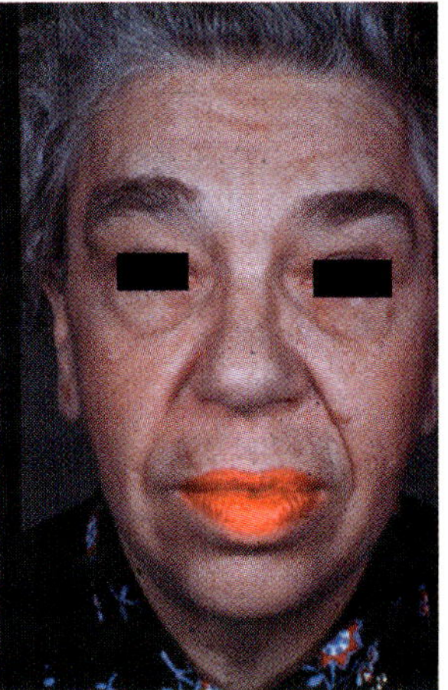

Figure MC-084
Coarsening of facial features and an enlarged jaw.

Text Links:
UCV2 **MC-084**
UCV1 BC-003

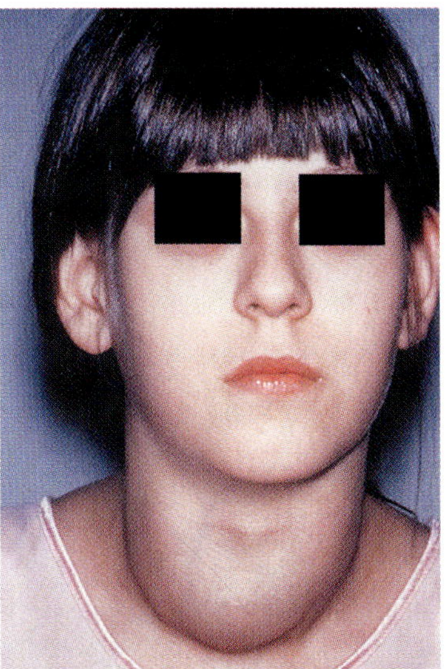

Figure MC-090A
Symmetrically enlarged anterior neck mass (goiter).

Text Links:
UCV2 **MC-090**
UCV1 BC-014

Figure MC-090B
Bilateral exophthalmos and conjunctival congestion.

Text Links:
UCV2 **MC-090**
UCV1 BC-014

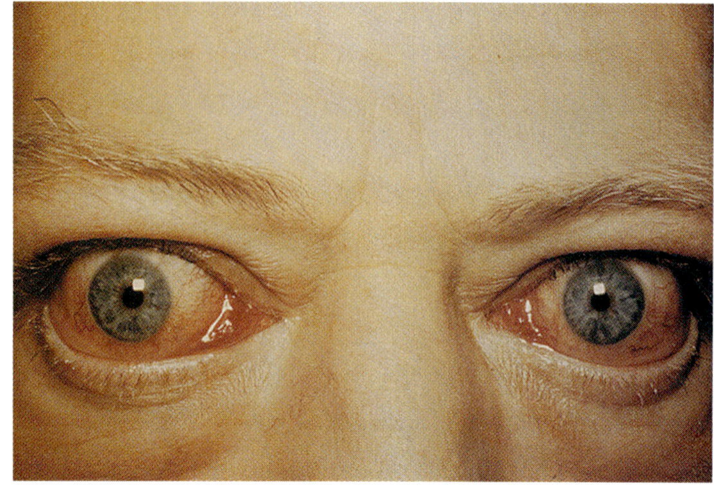

Figure MC-131
Inflamed papules, pustules, and closed comedones.

Text Link:
UCV2 **MC-131**

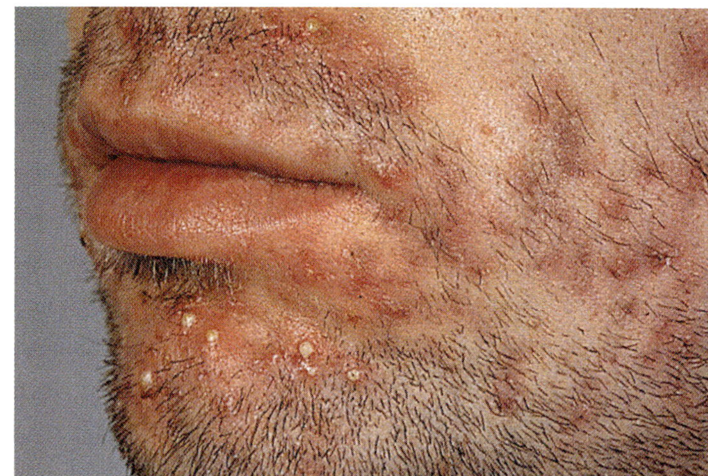

Figure MC-134
Discoid scarring alopecia with central atrophy and surrounding hyperpigmentation.

Text Link:
UCV2 **MC-134**

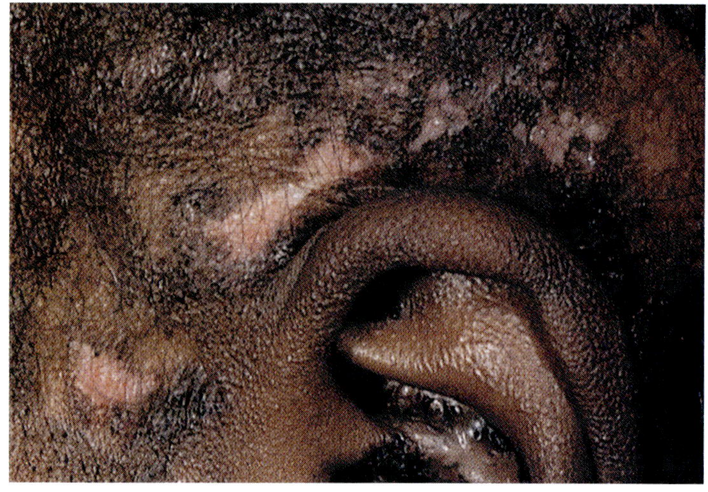

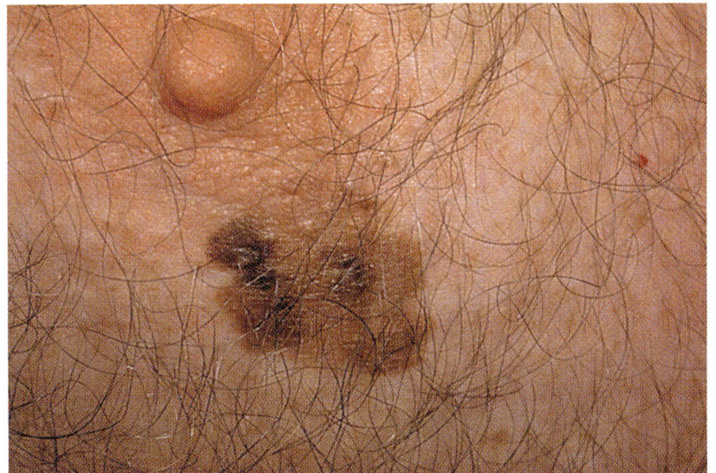

Figure MC-135
Asymmetric macule with irregular borders, variable color changes, and larger than 6 mm.

Text Links:
UCV2 **MC-135**
UCV1 P1-034

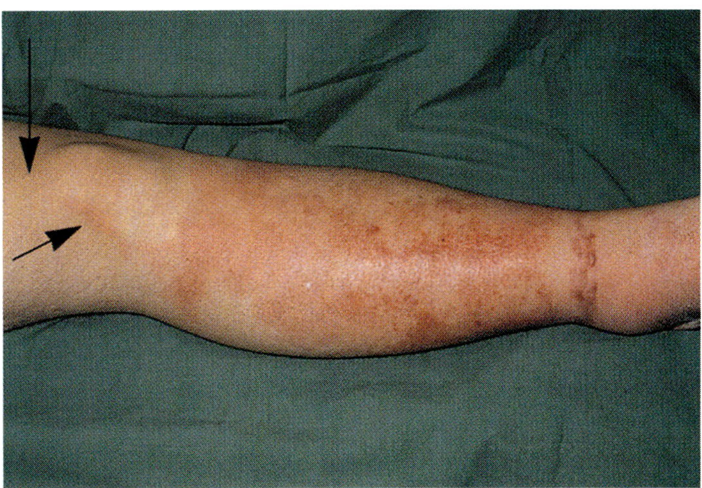

Figure MC-136
Sharply defined erythema with lymphangitic streak (arrows).

Text Links:
UCV2 **MC-136**
UCV1 M1-007

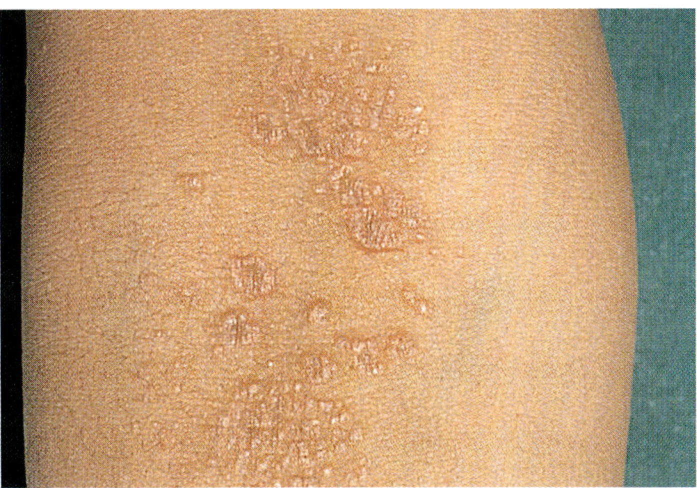

Figure MC-142
Persistently pruritic purplish, plane topped, polygonal papules with superficial white scale.

Text Links:
UCV2 **MC-142**
UCV1 P1-039

Figure MC-143
Flesh-colored nodules with a mosaic surface and central umbilication.

Text Links:
UCV2 **MC-143**
UCV1 M1-011

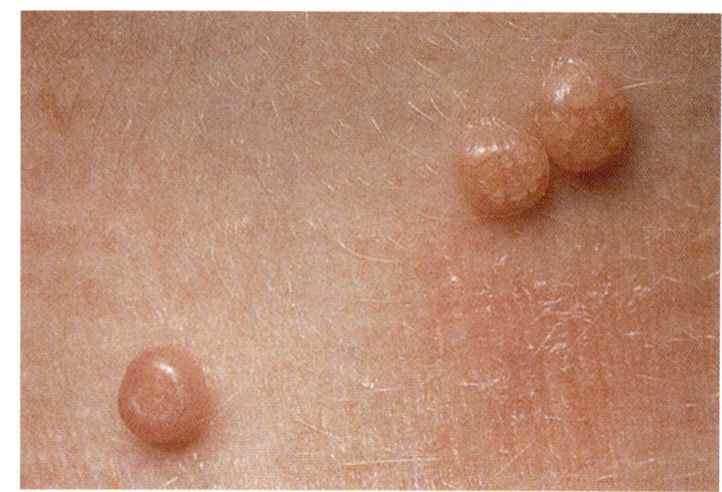

Figure MC-144
Generalized, well-demarcated, geographic, erythematous plaques (erythroderma).

Text Links:
UCV2 **MC-144**
UCV1 P1-041

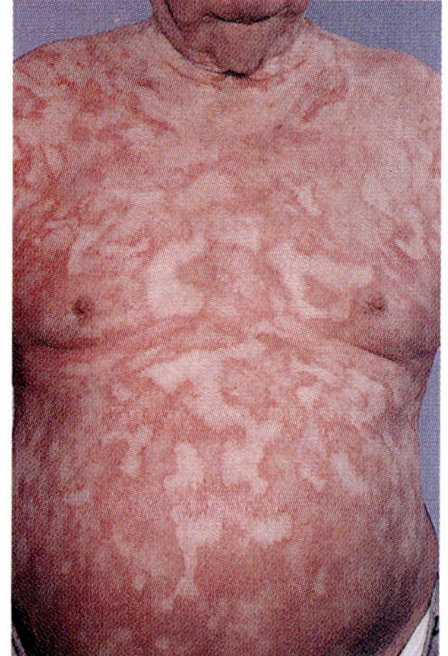

Figure MC-145
Multiple telangiectasias on the tongue.

Text Links:
UCV2 **MC-145**
UCV1 P1-042

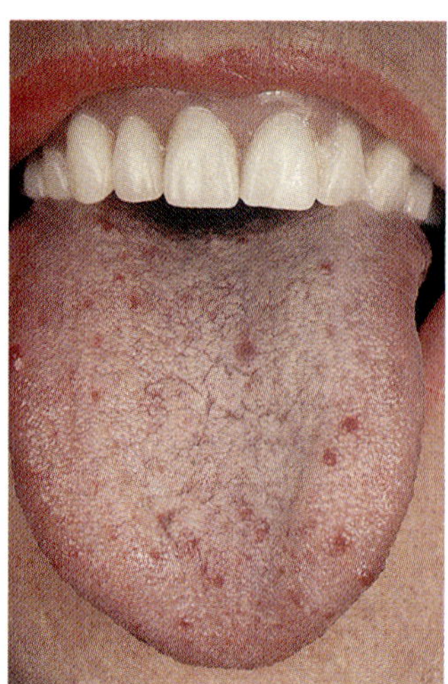

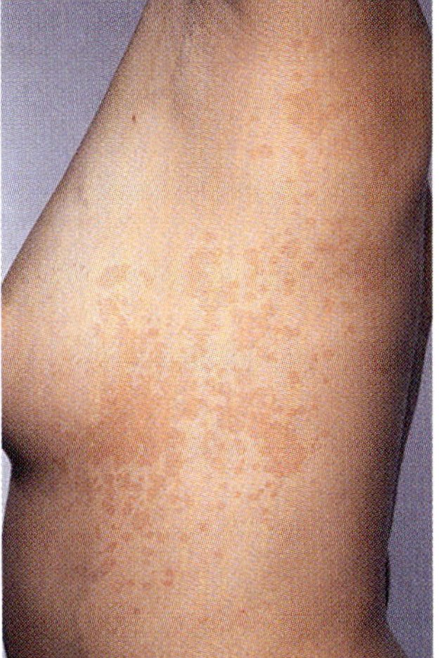

Figure MC-148
Tan brown, well-demarcated patches with fine scales on the trunk.

Text Links:
UCV2 **MC-148**
UCV1 M1-012

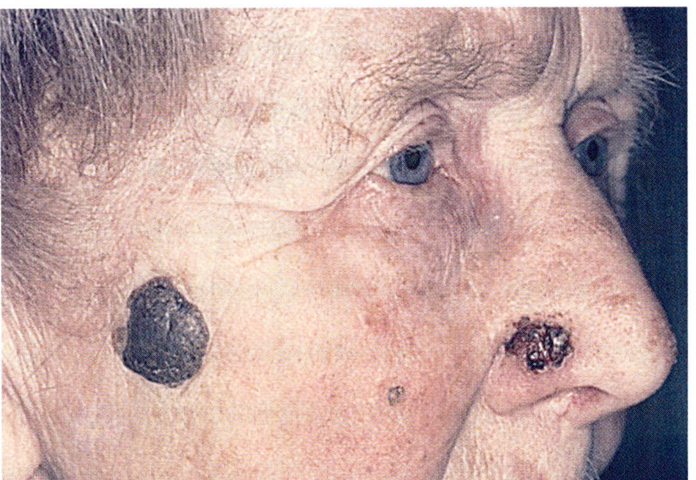

Figure MC-150
Brown verrucous plaque with a "stuck-on" appearance.

Text Link:
UCV2 **MC-150**

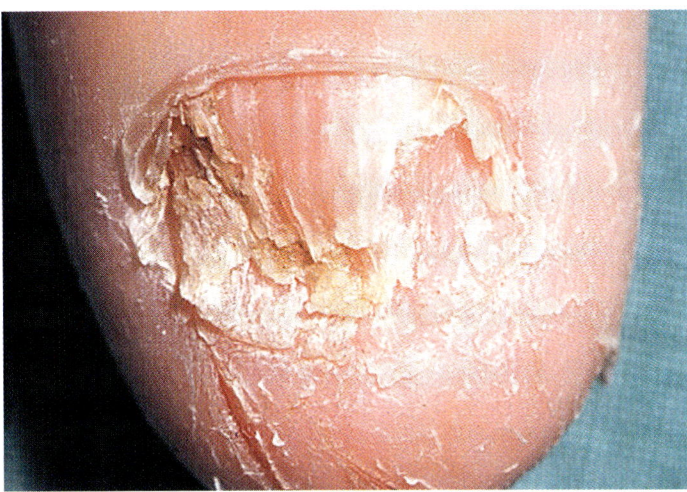

Figure MC-151
Nail dystrophy and subungual hyperkeratosis (onychomycosis).

Text Links:
UCV2 **MC-151**
UCV1 M1-015

Figure MC-153
Sharply defined, bilaterally symmetrical patches of depigmentation on the dorsum of the hands.

Text Links:
UCV2 **MC-153**
UCV1 P1-048

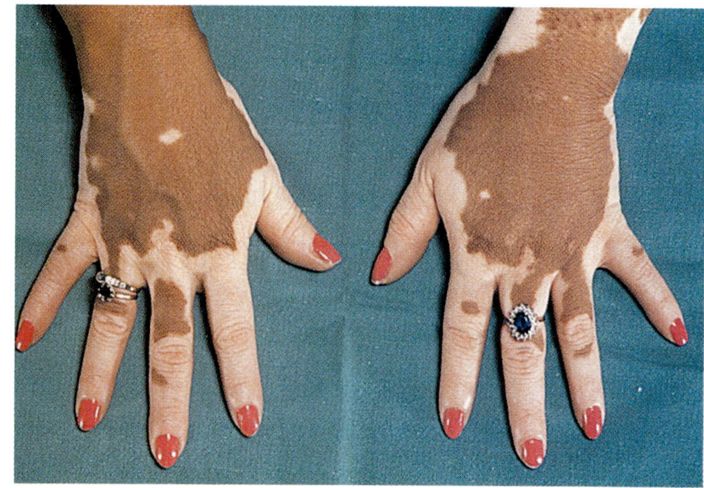

Figure MC-160
Isolated violaceous nodule.

Text Link:
UCV2 **MC-160**

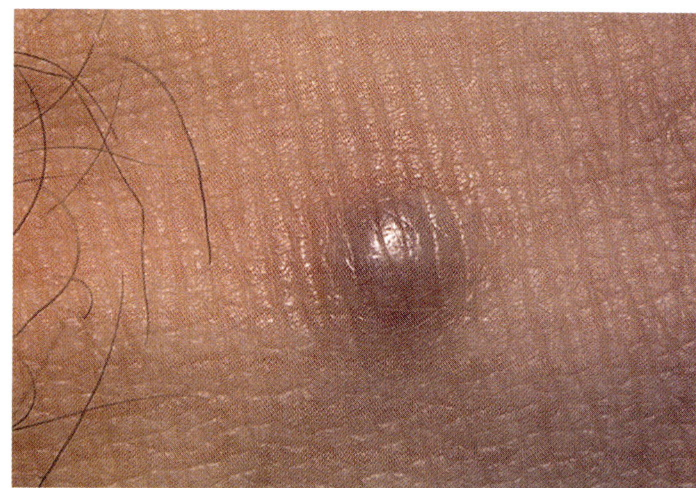

Figure MC-165
Multiple palmar vesicles.

Text Link:
UCV2 **MC-165**

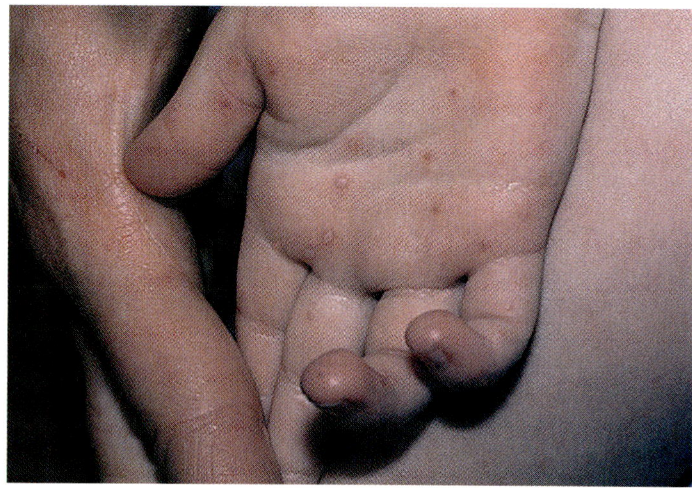

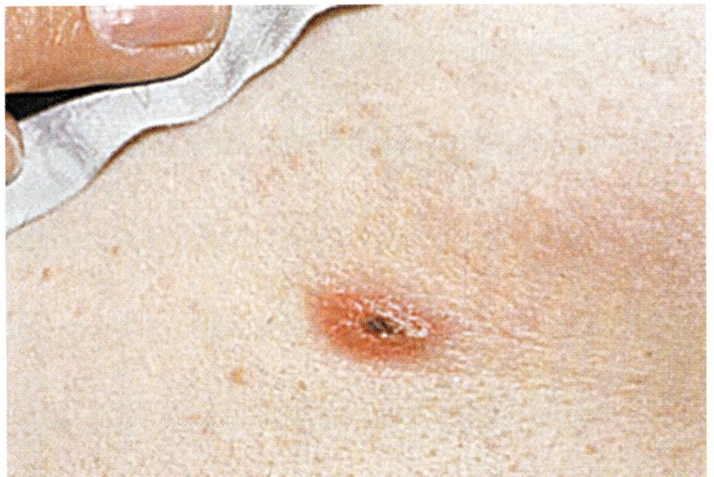

Figure MC-169
Erythematous macule with central black eschar.

Text Links:
UCV2 **MC-169**
UCV1 M1-086

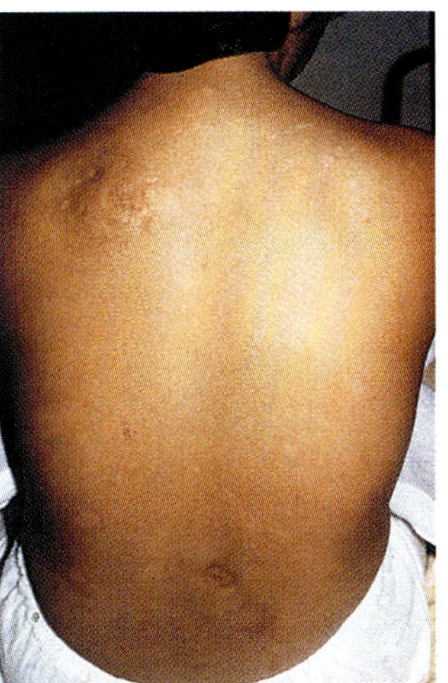

Figure MC-179A
Multiple plaques, nodules and hypopigmented patches.

Text Links:
UCV2 **MC-179**
UCV1 M2-015

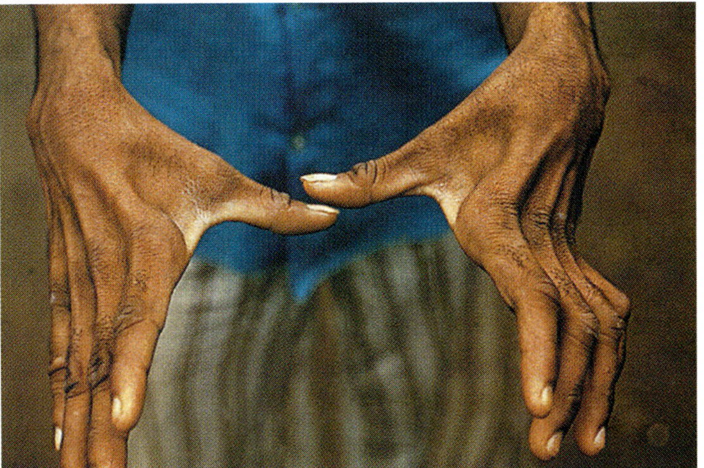

Figure MC-179B
Muscular atrophy and claw hand deformity secondary to bilateral ulnar nerve palsy.

Text Links:
UCV2 **MC-179**
UCV1 M2-016

Figure MC-186
Excoriated papules in interdigital web spaces.

Text Links:
UCV2 **MC-186**
UCV1 M2-049

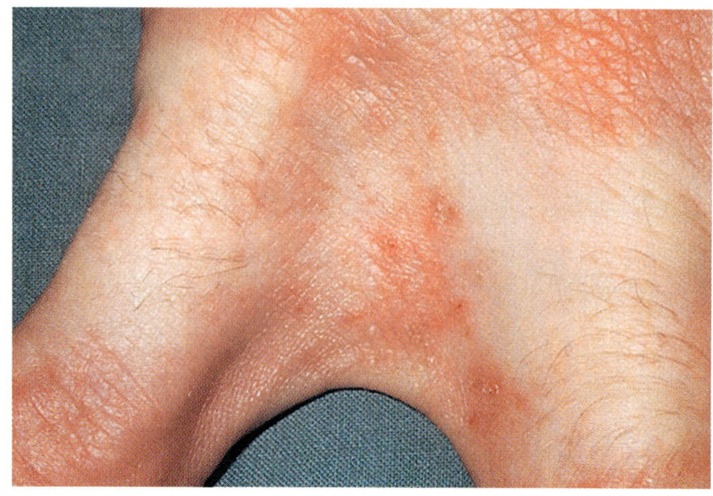

Figure MC-187A
Morbilliform erythematous rash on trunk (sandpaper rash).

Text Links:
UCV2 **MC-187**
UCV1 M2-050

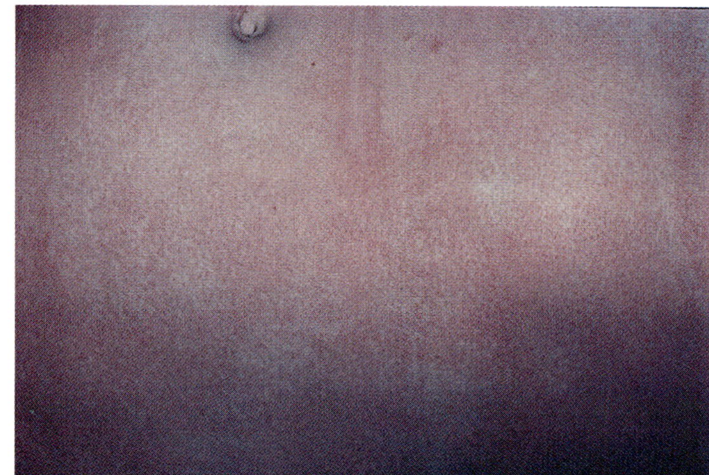

Figure MC-187B
Strawberry tongue.

Text Links:
UCV2 **MC-187**
UCV1 M2-050

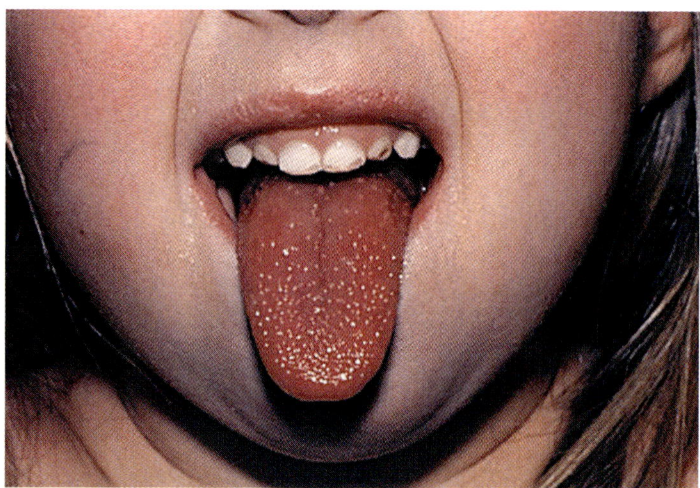

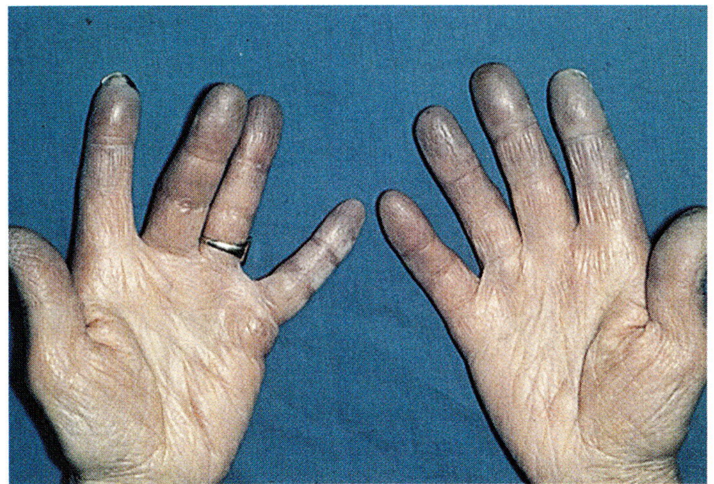

Figure MC-226
Bluish discoloration of the distal phalanges with signs of necrosis in the second digit.

Text Links:
UCV2 **MC-226**
UCV1 P3-089

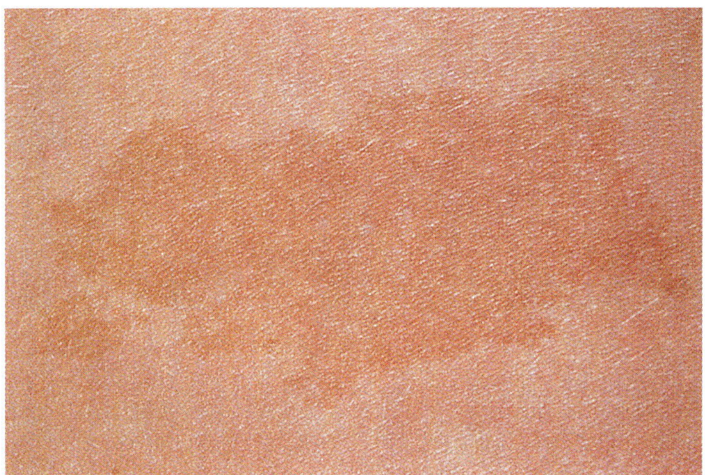

Figure MC-255A
Tan macule with ill-defined borders (café-au-lait spot).

Text Link:
UCV2 **MC-255**

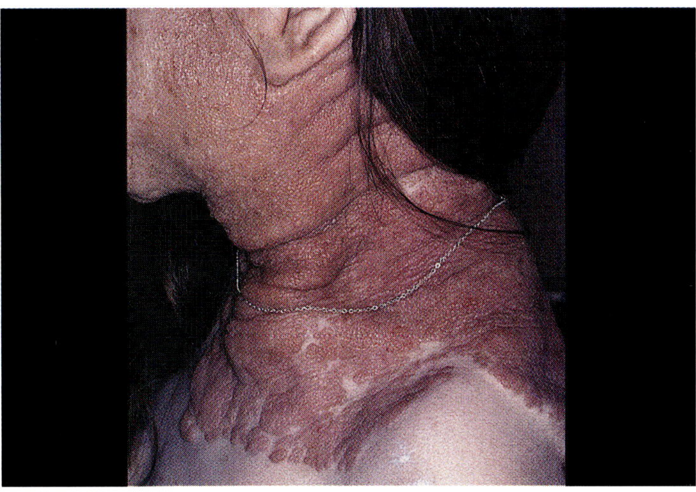

Figure MC-255B
Rubbery redish brown nodules and plaques (plexiform neurofibroma).

Text Link:
UCV2 **MC-255**

Figure MC-259
Well-demarcated, hemorrhagic ulcer on the sole, with exposed subcutaneous fat.

Text Links:
UCV2 **MC-259**
UCV1 P3-029

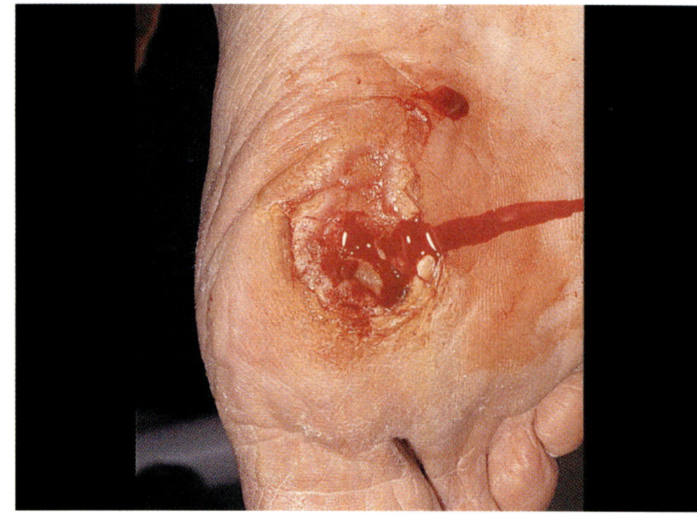

Figure MC-263
Large, hemorrhagic, pedunculated mass overlying thoracic spine.

Text Links:
UCV2 **MC-263**
UCV1 A-069

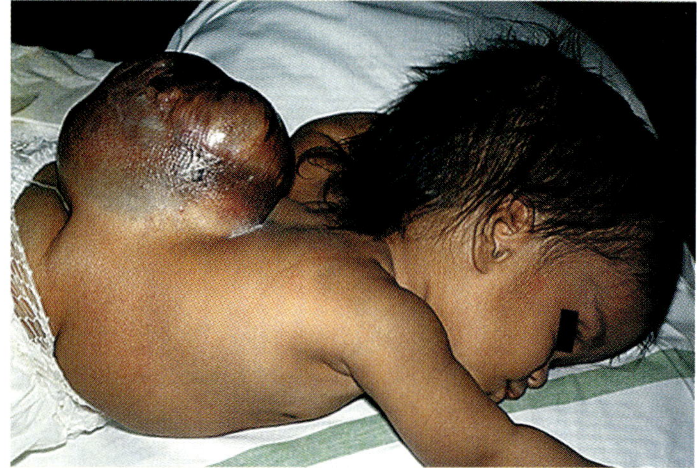

Figure MC-299
Bilateral bright malar erythema (slapped cheeks).

Text Links:
UCV2 **MC-299**
UCV1 M1-009

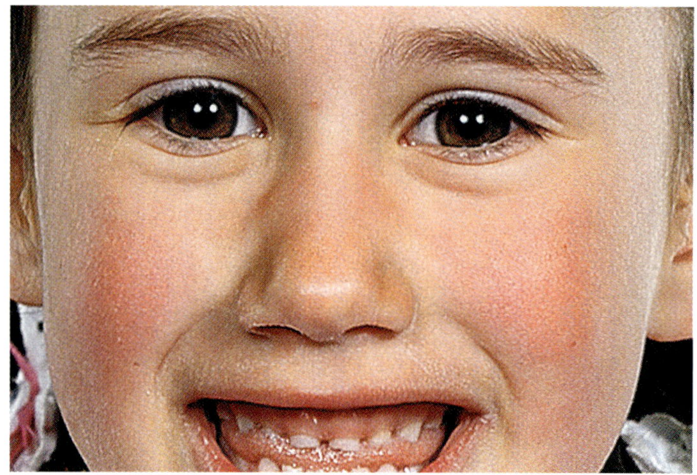

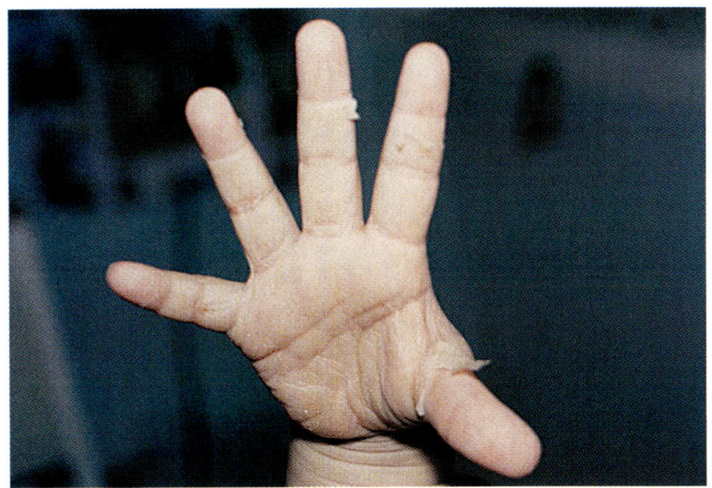

Figure MC-300
Palmar desquamation.

Text Links:
UCV2 **MC-300**
UCV1 P1-038

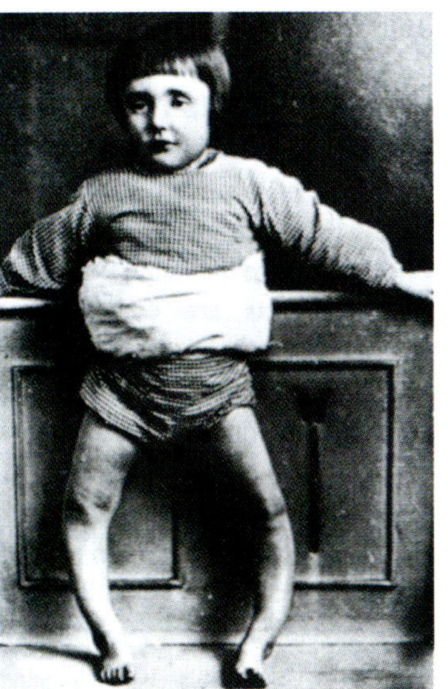

Figure MC-308
Frontal bossing and bowing of the femoral and tibial bones.

Text Links:
UCV2 **MC-308**
UCV1 BC-029

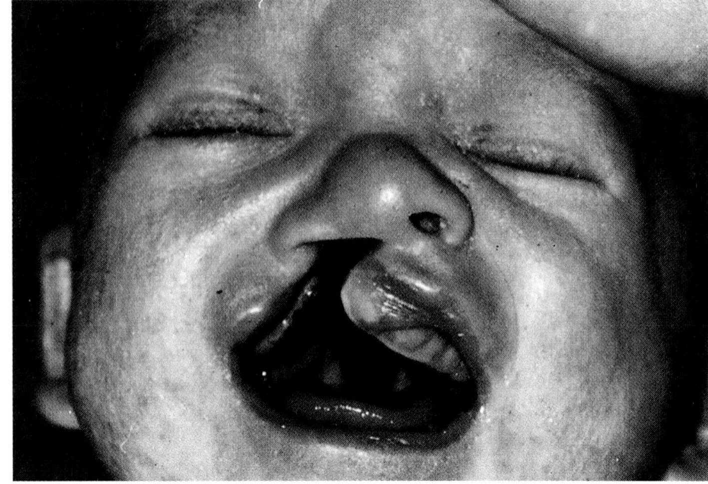

Figure MC-314A
Abnormal communication between the lip, the alveolar process of the maxilla, and the hard and soft palates.

Text Link:
UCV2 **MC-314**

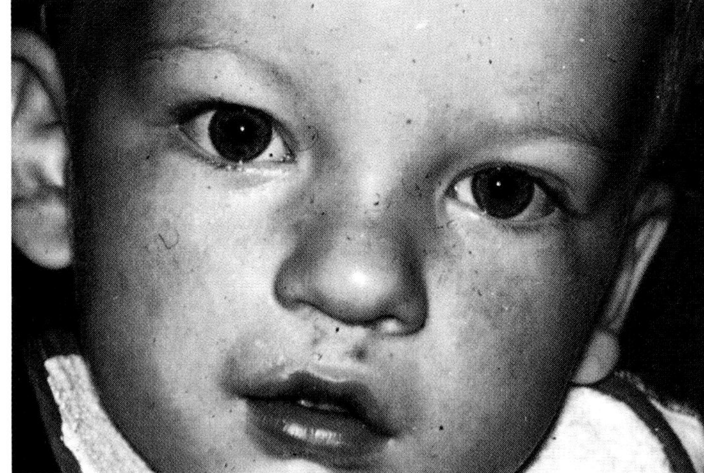

Figure MC-314B
Following facial reconstruction for cleft lip.

Text Link:
UCV2 **MC-314**

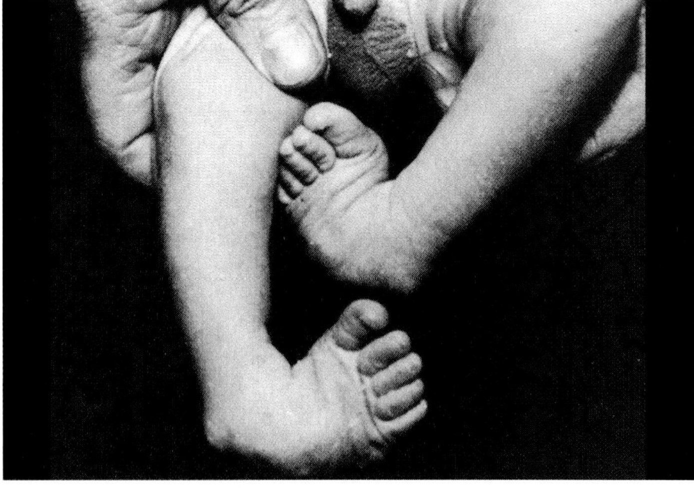

Figure MC-315
Club feet (talipes equino-varus).

Text Link:
UCV2 **MC-315**

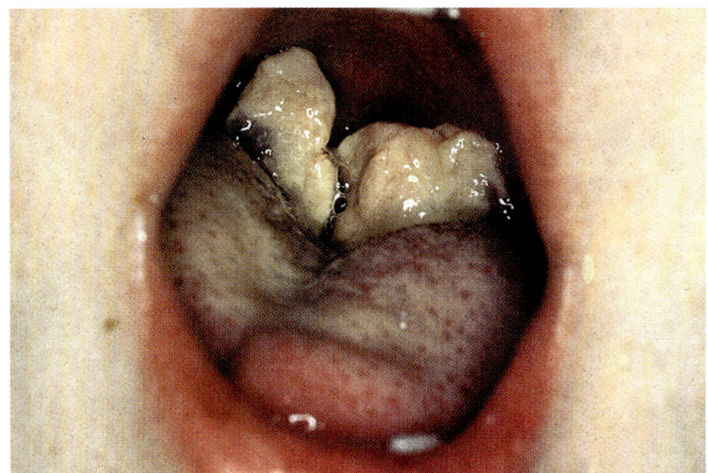

Figure MC-327
Thick, white-gray membrane loosely adherent to the tonsils and oropharynx (pseudomembrane).

Text Links:
UCV2 **MC-324**
UCV1 M1-082

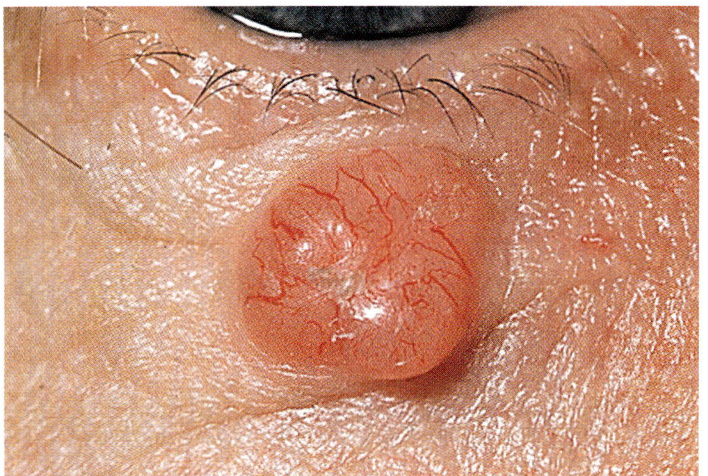

Figure MC-335A
Pearly papule with superficial telangiectasias and a rolled border.

Text Links:
UCV2 **MC-335**
UCV1 P1-031

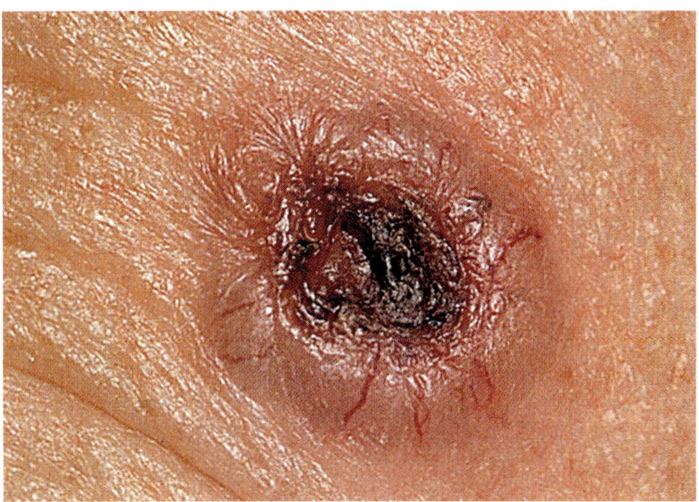

Figure MC-335B
Pearly papule with rolled borders and central ulceration.

Text Links:
UCV2 **MC-335**
UCV1 P1-031

Figure MC-349A
Supra-auricular vascular plaque.

Text Link:
UCV2 MC-349

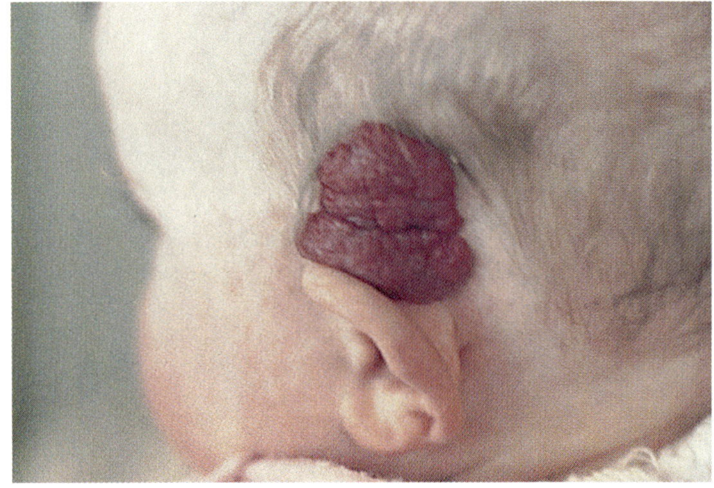

Figure MC-349B
Large vascular lesion arising from the forehead and obstructing the right eye.

Text Link:
UCV2 MC-349

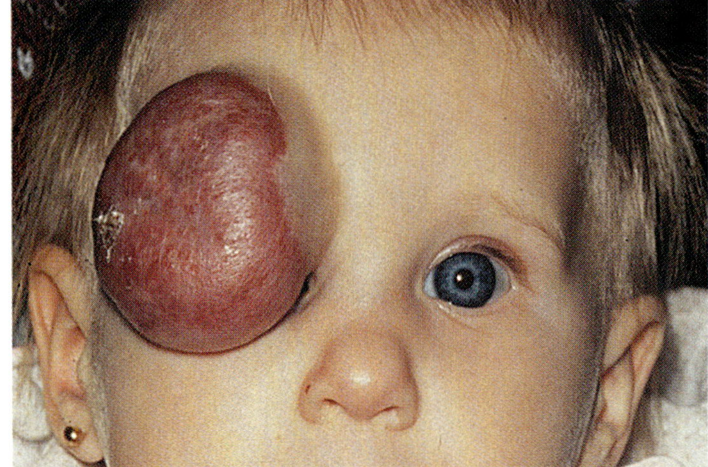

Figure MC-349C
Appearance following resection of the vascular lesion.

Text Link:
UCV2 MC-349

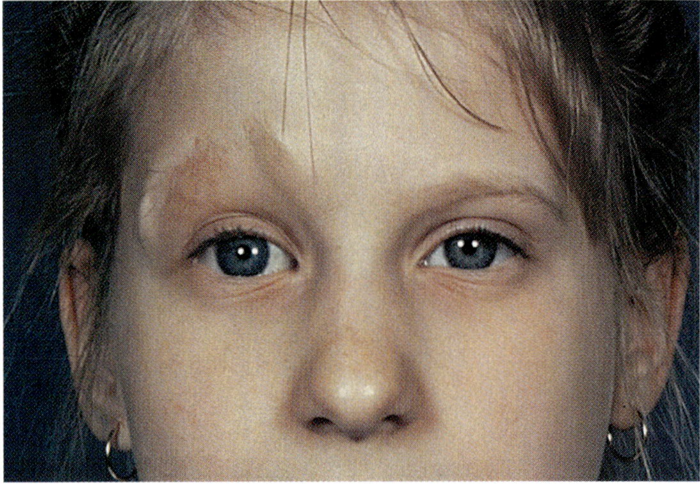

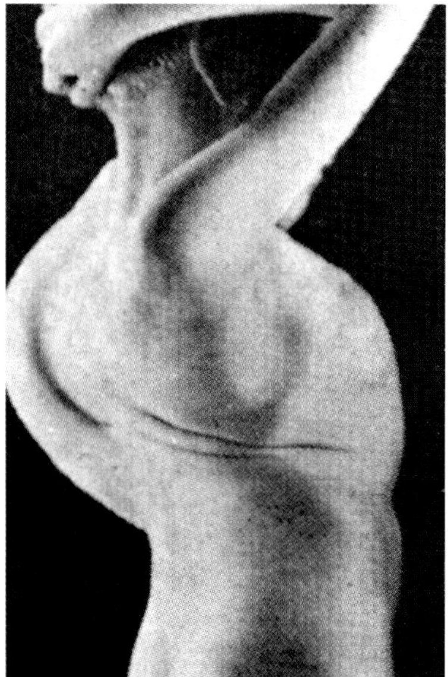

Figure MC-362A
Severe lateral curvature of the spine with left-sided thoracic convexity and posterior bulging of the ribs.

Text Link:
UCV2 **MC-362A**

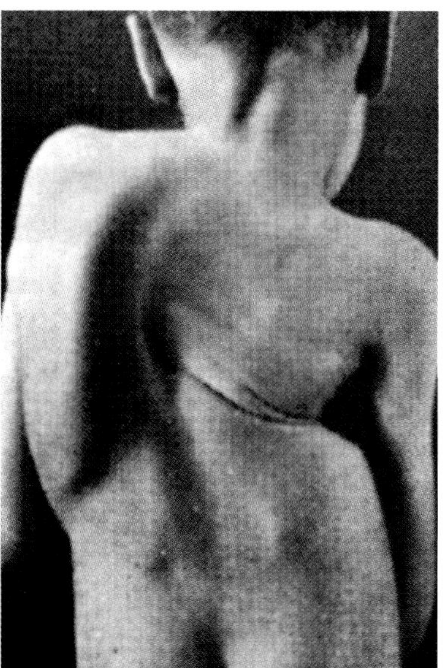

Figure MC-362B
Severe curvature of the spine with right-sided thoracic concavity and anterior displacement of the ribs.

Text Link:
UCV2 **MC-362**

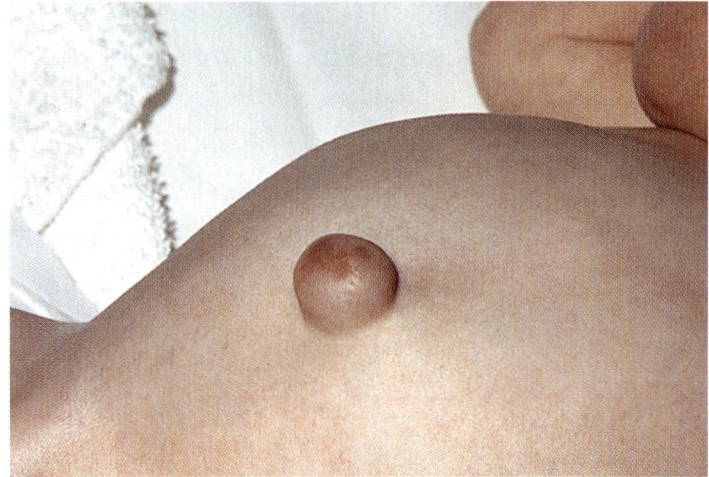

Figure MC-363A
Reducible midline abdominal mass protruding through the umbilicus of a newborn.

Text Link:
UCV2 **MC-363**

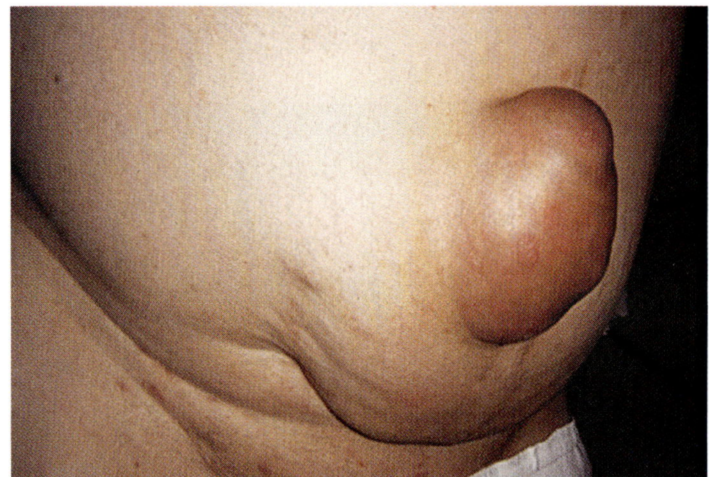

Figure MC-363B
Obese female with protuberant abdominal mass.

Text Link:
UCV2 **MC-363**

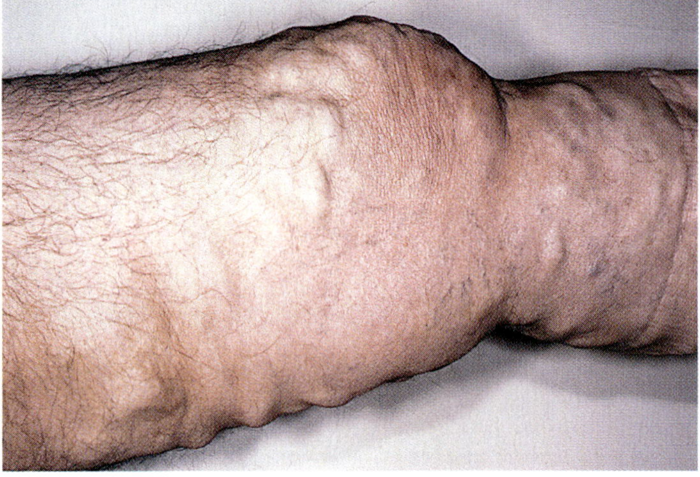

Figure MC-364
Dilated, tortuous veins on the lower extremity.

Text Links:
UCV2 **MC-364**
UCV1 A-041

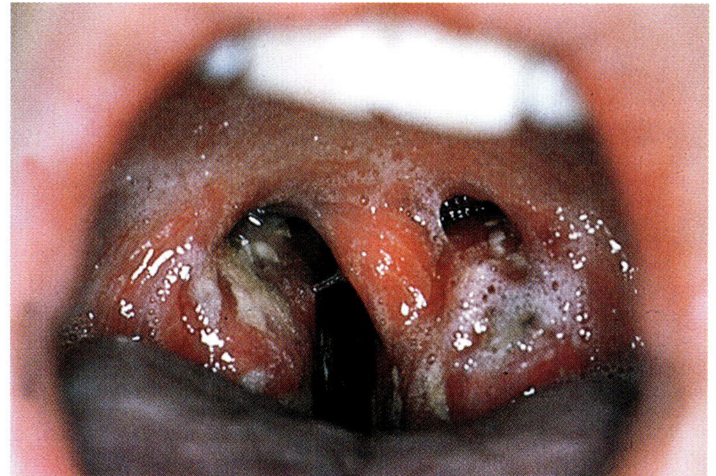

Figure Z-A-017
Enlarged, erythematous tonsils with purulent exudate and uvular deviation.

Text Link:
UCV1 A-017

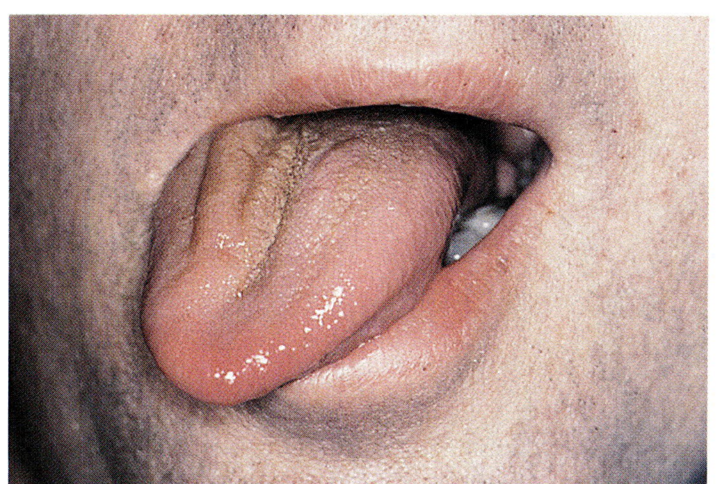

Figure Z-A-061
Lateral deviation of the tongue.

Text Link:
UCV1 A-061

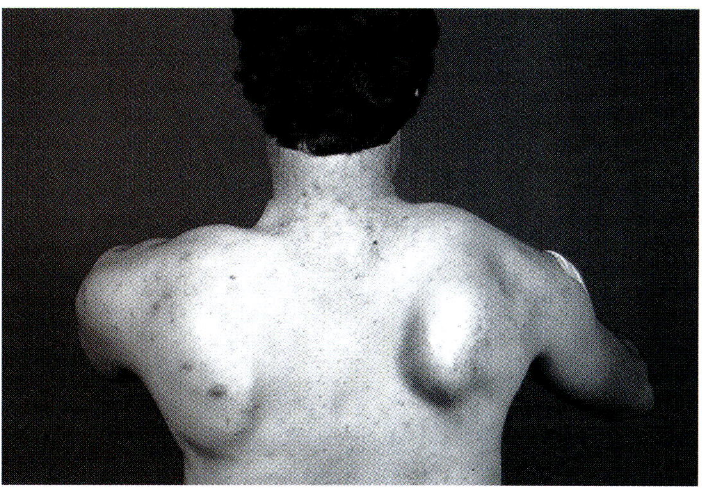

Figure Z-A-063
Protrusion and elevation (winging) of the right scapula.

Text Link:
UCV1 A-063

Figure Z-BC-058
Multiple skeletal abnormalities and a gargoyle-like facial appearance.

Text Link:
UCV1 BC-058

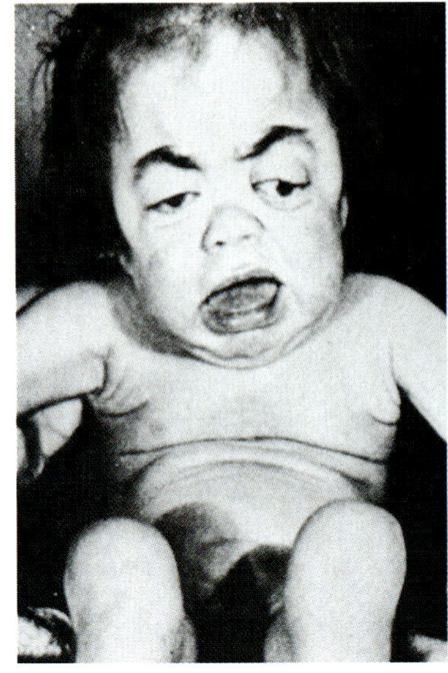

Figure Z-M1-054
Diffuse, erythematous maculopapular rash on the chest.

Text Link:
UCV1 M1-054

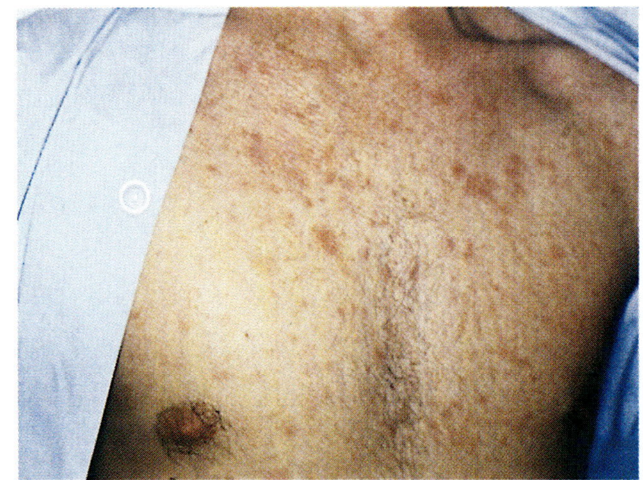

Figure Z-M1-096
Numerous red, well demarcated petechiae on upper extremity.

Text Link:
UCV1 M1-096B

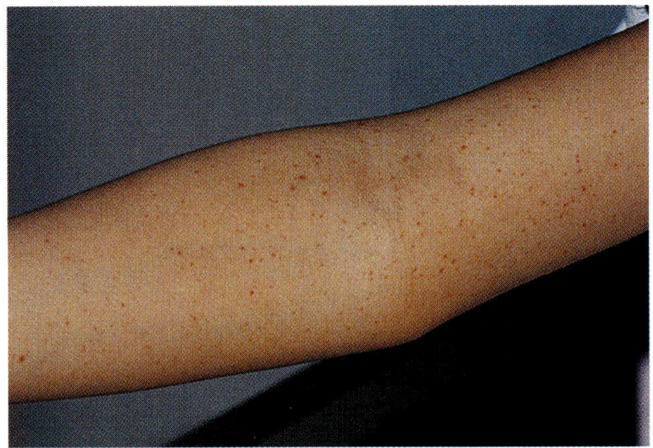

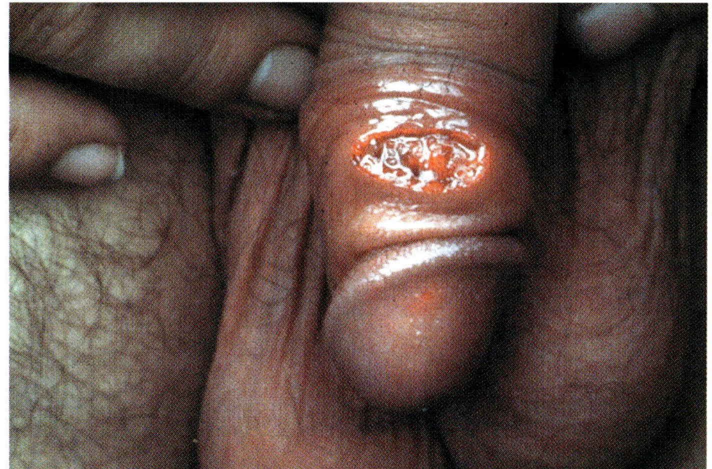

Figure Z-M2-059
Well-demarcated "punched out" painless ulcer on under side of foreskin (chancre).

Text Link:
UCV1 M2-059

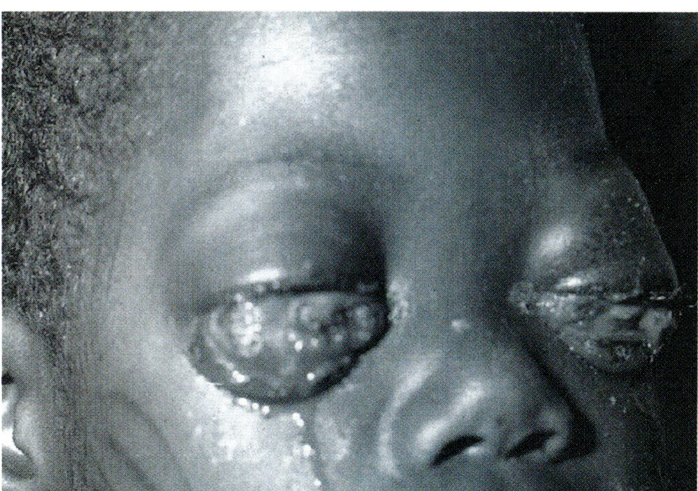

Figure Z-P2-018
Bilateral infiltration of the soft tissues and orbital bones.

Text Link:
UCV1 P2-018

MASTER CASE INDEX

Case Name	SER	BOOK	SubSpecialty	Case Number
Acute Conjunctivitis	UCV-1	MICRO-1	ENT/Ophthalmology	17
Acute Cystitis	UCV-1	MICRO-2	Nephrology/Urology	80
Acute Fatty Liver of Pregnancy	MC	OB/GYN	Obstetrics	290
Acute Intermittent Porphyria	MC	ER	Genetics	54
Acute Intermittent Porphyria	UCV-1	BIOCHEM	Genetics	42
Acute Lymphocytic Leukemia (ALL)	UCV-1	PATHOPHYS-2	Hematology/Oncology	13
Acute Lymphocytic Leukemia (ALL)	UCV-2	PED	Hematology/Oncology	16
Acute Myelogenous Leukemia (AML)	UCV-1	PATHOPHYS-2	Hematology/Oncology	14
Acute Myelogenous Leukemia (AML)	UCV-2	IM-1	Hematology/Oncology	41
Acute Renal Failure—Prerenal	MC	ER	Nephrology/Urology	59
Acute Rheumatic Fever	UCV-1	MICRO-1	Infectious Disease	52
Acute Rheumatic Fever	UCV-2	PED	Infectious Disease	25
Acute Sinusitis	MC	ER	ENT/Ophthalmology	29
Acute Sinusitis	UCV-1	MICRO-1	ENT/Ophthalmology	18
Acute Torticollis	UCV-1	ANAT	Neurology	50
Acute Tubular Necrosis—Ischemic	UCV-2	IM-2	Nephrology/Urology	32
Acute Tubular Necrosis—Toxic	UCV-2	IM-2	Nephrology/Urology	33
Acute Tubular Necrosis (ATN)	UCV-1	PATHOPHYS-2	Nephrology/Urology	48
Addison's Disease	UCV-1	BIOCHEM	Endocrinology	4
Addison's Disease	UCV-2	IM-1	Endocrinology	16
Adjustment Disorder	UCV-1	BEHAV-SC	Adjustment Disorders	26
Adjustment Disorder	UCV-2	PSYCH	Adjustment Disorders	4
Adnexal Torsion	MC	OB/GYN	Gynecology	272
Adult Polycystic Kidney Disease	MC	IM-2	Nephrology/Urology	196
Adult Polycystic Kidney Disease (APKD)	UCV-1	PATHOPHYS-2	Nephrology/Urology	49
Adult Respiratory Distress Syndrome (ARDS)	UCV-1	PATHOPHYS-2	Pulmonary	74
Adult Respiratory Distress Syndrome(ARDS)	UCV-2	IM-2	Pulmonary	42
Advance Directives	UCV-2	PSYCH	Ethics	29
Aflatoxin Carcinogenicity	UCV-1	PHARM	Toxicology	93
African Trypanosomiasis	UCV-1	MICRO-1	Infectious Disease	53
Agoraphobia	UCV-2	PSYCH	Anxiety Disorders	5
AIDS—Pediatric	UCV-2	PED	Infectious Disease	26
AIDS Dementia	UCV-1	BEHAV-SC	Neurology	1
AIDS-Related Complex (ARC)	UCV-1	MICRO-1	Infectious Disease	54
Albinism	UCV-1	BIOCHEM	Genetics	43
Alcohol Intoxication	MC	IM-2	Psychopharmacology	206

Case Name	SER	BOOK	SubSpecialty	Case Number
Alcoholic Hallucinosis	UCV-1	BEHAV-SC	Psychopharmacology	96
Alcoholic Ketoacidosis	MC	IM-2	Psychopharmacology	207
Alcoholism	UCV-1	PATHOPHYS-3	Psychopharmacology	78
Alcoholism	UCV-2	PSYCH	Psychopharmacology	17
Alkaptonuria	MC	PED	Genetics	316
Alkaptonuria	UCV-1	BIOCHEM	Genetics	44
Allergic Rhinitis (Hay Fever)	UCV-1	MICRO-1	ENT/Ophthalmology	19
Alpha-1-Antitrypsin Deficiency	UCV-1	BIOCHEM	Pulmonary	92
Alport's Disease	MC	PED	Nephrology/Urology	333
Alport's Disease	UCV-1	PATHOPHYS-2	Nephrology/Urology	50
Alternative Pharmacotherapy	UCV-1	PHARM	Gastroenterology	23
Aluminum Toxicity	UCV-1	PHARM	Toxicology	94
Amantadine Toxicity	UCV-1	PHARM	Neurology	62
Amebiasis	MC	IM-2	Infectious Disease	158
Amebic Colitis	UCV-1	MICRO-1	Infectious Disease	55
Amebic Liver Abscess	UCV-1	MICRO-1	Infectious Disease	56
Amebic Liver Abscess	UCV-2	IM-2	Infectious Disease	12
Amebic Meningoencephalitis	UCV-1	MICRO-1	Infectious Disease	57
Amiodarone Side Effects	UCV-1	PHARM	Cardiology	1
Ammonia Overdose	UCV-1	PHARM	Toxicology	95
Amnesia—Postencephalitis	UCV-1	BEHAV-SC	Neurology	2
Amniotic Fluid Embolism	UCV-2	OB/GYN	Obstetrics	34
Amphetamine Abuse	UCV-1	PHARM	Psychopharmacology	72
Amphetamine Toxicity	UCV-2	ER	Psychopharmacology	39
Amphetamine Withdrawal	UCV-1	PHARM	Psychopharmacology	73
Amphotericin B Toxicity	UCV-1	PHARM	Infectious Disease	45
Amyloidosis	MC	IM-2	Nephrology/Urology	197
Amyloidosis—Primary	UCV-1	PATHOPHYS-2	Nephrology/Urology	51
Amyotrophic Lateral Sclerosis (ALS)	UCV-1	PATHOPHYS-3	Neurology	1
Amyotrophic Lateral Sclerosis (ALS)	UCV-2	NEURO	Neurology	1
Anabolic Steroid Abuse	UCV-1	PHARM	Endocrinology	14
Anal Fissure	UCV-2	SURG	General Surgery	18
Anal Fistula	UCV-2	SURG	General Surgery	19
Anaphylaxis	UCV-1	MICRO-2	Immunology	1
Anaphylaxis	UCV-2	ER	Immunology	28
Anemia—Aplastic	MC	IM-1	Hematology/Oncology	114
Anemia—Aplastic	UCV-1	PATHOPHYS-2	Hematology/Oncology	15
Anemia—Aplastic Crisis (Parvovirus B19)	UCV-1	MICRO-1	Hematology/Oncology	46

Case Name	SER	BOOK	SubSpecialty	Case Number
Anemia—Autoimmune Hemolytic	MC	IM-1	Hematology/Oncology	115
Anemia—Autoimmune Hemolytic	UCV-1	PATHOPHYS-2	Hematology/Oncology	16
Anemia—*Diphyllobothrium latum*	UCV-1	MICRO-1	Hematology/Oncology	47
Anemia—Folate Deficiency	MC	IM-1	Hematology/Oncology	116
Anemia—Folate Deficiency	UCV-1	BIOCHEM	Hematology/Oncology	75
Anemia—Iron Deficiency	UCV-1	BIOCHEM	Hematology/Oncology	76
Anemia—Iron Deficiency	UCV-2	IM-1	Hematology/Oncology	42
Anemia—Iron Deficiency	UCV-2	OB/GYN	Obstetrics	35
Anemia—Vitamin B_{12} Deficiency	UCV-1	BIOCHEM	Hematology/Oncology	77
Anemia—Vitamin B_{12} Deficiency	UCV-2	IM-1	Hematology/Oncology	43
Anemia of Chronic Disease	MC	IM-1	Hematology/Oncology	117
Anemia of Pregnancy	UCV-2	OB/GYN	Obstetrics	36
Aniline Dye Carcinogenicity	UCV-1	PHARM	Hematology/Oncology	33
Ankle Sprain	UCV-1	ANAT	Orthopedics	76
Ankylosing Spondylitis	UCV-1	PATHOPHYS-3	Rheumatology	79
Ankylosing Spondylitis	UCV-2	IM-2	Rheumatology	50
Anorectic/Anti-obesity Agents	UCV-1	PHARM	Gastroenterology	24
Anorexia Nervosa	UCV-1	BEHAV-SC	Eating Disorders	45
Anorexia Nervosa	UCV-2	PSYCH	Eating Disorders	27
Antabuse Effect	UCV-1	BIOCHEM	Psychopharmacology	90
Anthrax	UCV-1	MICRO-1	Infectious Disease	58
Anticonvulsant Osteomalacia	UCV-1	PHARM	Neurology	63
Antiphospholipid Antibody Syndrome	MC	IM-1	Hematology/Oncology	118
Antiphospholipid Antibody Syndrome	UCV-1	PATHOPHYS-2	Hematology/Oncology	17
Antisocial Personality Disorder	UCV-1	BEHAV-SC	Personality Disorders	66
Antisocial Personality Disorder	UCV-2	PSYCH	Personality Disorders	44
Aortic Dissection	UCV-1	PATHOPHYS-1	Cardiology	1
Aortic Dissection	UCV-2	ER	Cardiology	1
Aortic Insufficiency	UCV-1	PATHOPHYS-1	Cardiology	2
Aortic Insufficiency	UCV-2	IM-1	Cardiology	1
Aortic Stenosis	UCV-1	PATHOPHYS-1	Cardiology	3
Aortic Stenosis	UCV-2	IM-1	Cardiology	2
Aphasia—Broca's	UCV-1	PATHOPHYS-3	Neurology	2
Aphasia—Conduction	MC	NEURO	Neurology	233
Aphasia—Wernicke's	UCV-1	ANAT	Neurology	51
Appendicitis	UCV-1	PATHOPHYS-2	General Surgery	3
Appendicitis—Acute	UCV-2	SURG	General Surgery	20
Appetite Stimulants—Megestrol/THC	UCV-1	PHARM	Gastroenterology	25

Case Name	SER	BOOK	SubSpecialty	Case Number
Arm—Radial Nerve Palsy	UCV-1	ANAT	Orthopedics	77
Arsenic Poisoning	UCV-1	PHARM	Toxicology	96
Arteriovenous Fistula	UCV-1	ANAT	Cardiology	1
Asbestosis	UCV-1	PATHOPHYS-2	Pulmonary	75
Asbestosis	UCV-2	IM-2	Pulmonary	43
Ascending Cholangitis	UCV-1	PATHOPHYS-1	Gastroenterology	76
Ascending Cholangitis	UCV-2	ER	Gastroenterology	13
Aspergillosis	MC	IM-2	Infectious Disease	159
Aspergillosis	UCV-1	MICRO-1	Infectious Disease	59
Aspergillosis—Allergic	UCV-2	IM-2	Infectious Disease	13
Aspergillosis—Allergic Bronchopulmonary	UCV-1	MICRO-1	Infectious Disease	60
Aspiration Pneumonia with Lung Abscess	UCV-1	MICRO-1	Infectious Disease	61
Asthma	UCV-1	PATHOPHYS-2	Pulmonary	76
Asthma—Atopic	UCV-2	PED	Pulmonary	54
Asthma—Severe Acute	UCV-1	PHARM	Pulmonary	90
Asthma—Severe Acute	UCV-2	ER	Pulmonary	45
Asthma, Chronic	UCV-2	IM-2	Pulmonary	44
Astrocytoma	UCV-1	ANAT	Neurology	52
Astrocytoma	UCV-2	NEURO	Neurology	2
Asystole	MC	ER	Cardiology	1
Atelectasis—Postoperative	UCV-1	PATHOPHYS-2	Pulmonary	77
Atherosclerosis	UCV-1	PATHOPHYS-1	Cardiology	4
Atopic Dermatitis	MC	IM-2	Dermatology	132
Atopic Dermatitis	UCV-1	PATHOPHYS-1	Dermatology	30
Atopy	MC	IM-2	Immunology	194
Atrial Fibrillation	MC	IM-1	Cardiology	74
Atrial Fibrillation	UCV-1	PATHOPHYS-1	Cardiology	5
Atrial Flutter	MC	IM-1	Cardiology	75
Atrial Myxoma	UCV-1	PATHOPHYS-1	Cardiology	6
Atrial Myxoma	UCV-2	IM-1	Cardiology	3
Atrial Septal Defect	UCV-1	ANAT	Cardiology	2
Atrial Septal Defect	UCV-2	SURG	Cardiology	1
Attention-Deficit Hyperactivity Disorder	UCV-1	BEHAV-SC	Child Psychiatry	32
Attention-Deficit Hyperactivity Disorder	UCV-2	PSYCH	Child	11
Atypical Mycobacterial Infection	UCV-1	MICRO-1	Infectious Disease	62
Autism	UCV-1	BEHAV-SC	Child Psychiatry	33
Autism	UCV-2	PSYCH	Child	12

	Case Name	SER	BOOK	SubSpecialty	Case Number
	AV Malformation	MC	IM-1	General Surgery	113
	Avoidant Personality Disorder	UCV-1	BEHAV-SC	Personality Disorders	67
B	Bacillary Angiomatosis	MC	IM-2	Infectious Disease	160
	Bacillus cereus Food Poisoning	UCV-1	MICRO-1	Infectious Disease	63
	Bacterial Vaginosis	UCV-1	MICRO-2	Gynecology	101
	Bacterial Vaginosis	UCV-2	OB/GYN	Gynecology	1
	Baker's Cyst	MC	IM-2	Rheumatology	217
	Barbiturate Intoxication	UCV-1	PHARM	Psychopharmacology	74
	Barrett's Esophagus	MC	IM-1	Gastroenterology	98
	Barrett's Esophagus	UCV-1	PATHOPHYS-1	Gastroenterology	77
	Bartonellosis	UCV-1	MICRO-1	Infectious Disease	64
	Bartter's Syndrome	MC	IM-1	Endocrinology	85
	Bartter's Syndrome	UCV-1	BIOCHEM	Endocrinology	5
	Basal Cell Carcinoma	MC	SURG	Dermatology	335
	Basal Cell Carcinoma	UCV-1	PATHOPHYS-1	Dermatology	31
	Bee Sting	MC	IM-2	Immunology	195
	Behçet's Disease	MC	IM-2	Rheumatology	218
	Bell's Palsy	UCV-1	ANAT	Neurology	53
	Bell's Palsy	UCV-2	NEURO	Neurology	3
	Benign Positional Vertigo	MC	ER	ENT/Ophthalmology	30
	Benign Positional Vertigo	UCV-1	PATHOPHYS-1	ENT/Ophthalmology	63
	Benign Prostatic Hypertrophy (BPH)	UCV-1	PATHOPHYS-2	Nephrology/Urology	52
	Benign Prostatic Hypertrophy (BPH)	UCV-2	SURG	Nephrology/Urology	35
	Bereavement	UCV-2	PSYCH	Mood Disorders	39
	Bernard–Soulier Syndrome	MC	IM-1	Hematology/Oncology	119
	Beta-Blocker Overdose	UCV-1	PHARM	Cardiology	2
	Bipolar I Disorder, Manic Type	UCV-1	BEHAV-SC	Mood Disorders	50
	Bipolar I Disorder, Manic Type	UCV-2	PSYCH	Mood Disorders	40
	Bipolar II Mood Disorder	UCV-1	BEHAV-SC	Mood Disorders	51
	Bladder Cancer	UCV-1	PATHOPHYS-2	Nephrology/Urology	53
	Bladder Cancer	UCV-2	SURG	Nephrology/Urology	36
	Bladder Outlet Obstruction, Nephropathy	UCV-1	PATHOPHYS-2	Nephrology/Urology	54
	Blastomycosis	MC	IM-2	Infectious Disease	161
	Blastomycosis	UCV-1	MICRO-1	Infectious Disease	65
	Bleomycin Toxicity	UCV-1	PHARM	Hematology/Oncology	34
	Body Dysmorphic Disorder	UCV-1	BEHAV-SC	Somatoform Disorders	88
	Body Dysmorphic Disorder	UCV-2	PSYCH	Somatoform Disorders	50
	Boerhaave's Syndrome	MC	SURG	Gastroenterology	339

Case Name	SER	BOOK	SubSpecialty	Case Number
Boerhaave's Syndrome	UCV-1	ANAT	Gastroenterology	15
Borderline Personality Disorder	UCV-1	BEHAV-SC	Personality Disorders	68
Borderline Personality Disorder	UCV-2	PSYCH	Personality Disorders	45
Botulism	UCV-1	MICRO-1	Infectious Disease	66
Botulism	UCV-2	IM-2	Infectious Disease	14
Botulism—Infant	UCV-2	PED	Infectious Disease	27
Brain Abscess	MC	NEURO	Neurology	234
Brain Abscess	UCV-1	MICRO-2	Neurology	87
Breast—Cystosarcoma Phyllodes	MC	OB/GYN	Gynecology	273
Breast—Cystosarcoma Phyllodes	UCV-1	PATHOPHYS-3	Gynecology	36
Breast—Fat Necrosis	UCV-1	PATHOPHYS-3	Gynecology	37
Breast—Fibrocystic Disease	MC	OB/GYN	Gynecology	274
Breast—Fibrocystic Disease	UCV-1	PATHOPHYS-3	Gynecology	38
Breast—Inflammatory Carcinoma	UCV-1	PATHOPHYS-3	Gynecology	39
Breast—Intraductal Papilloma	UCV-1	PATHOPHYS-3	Gynecology	40
Breast—Intraductal Papilloma	UCV-2	OB/GYN	Gynecology	2
Breast—Lobular Carcinoma	UCV-1	PATHOPHYS-3	Gynecology	41
Breast—Paget's Disease	MC	OB/GYN	Gynecology	275
Breast—Paget's Disease	UCV-1	PATHOPHYS-3	Gynecology	42
Breast Abscess	MC	OB/GYN	Gynecology	276
Breast Abscess	UCV-1	MICRO-2	Gynecology	102
Breast Carcinoma	UCV-1	PATHOPHYS-3	Gynecology	43
Breast Carcinoma	UCV-2	OB/GYN	Gynecology	3
Breast Fibroadenoma	MC	OB/GYN	Gynecology	277
Breast Fibroadenoma	UCV-1	PATHOPHYS-3	Gynecology	44
Brief Psychotic Disorder	UCV-2	PSYCH	Psychotic Disorders	47
Brief Psychotic Episode	UCV-1	BEHAV-SC	Psychotic Disorders	77
Bronchiectasis	MC	IM-2	Pulmonary	208
Bronchiectasis	UCV-1	PATHOPHYS-2	Pulmonary	78
Brown-Séquard Syndrome	UCV-1	ANAT	Neurology	54
Brown-Séquard Syndrome	UCV-2	NEURO	Neurology	4
Brucellosis	MC	IM-2	Infectious Disease	162
Brucellosis	UCV-1	MICRO-1	Infectious Disease	67
Bruton's Agammaglobulinemia	UCV-2	PED	Immunology	36
Budd–Chiari Syndrome	MC	IM-1	Gastroenterology	99
Budd–Chiari Syndrome	UCV-1	PATHOPHYS-1	Gastroenterology	78
Bulimia Nervosa	UCV-1	BEHAV-SC	Eating Disorders	46
Bulimia Nervosa	UCV-2	PSYCH	Eating Disorders	28

	Case Name	SER	BOOK	SubSpecialty	Case Number
	Bullous Pemphigoid	MC	ER	Dermatology	17
	Burkitt's Lymphoma	UCV-1	PATHOPHYS-2	Hematology/Oncology	18
	Burkitt's Lymphoma	UCV-2	IM-1	Hematology/Oncology	44
C	C1 Spinal Cord Injury	UCV-1	PATHOPHYS-3	Neurology	3
	CAD—Myocardial Infarction	UCV-1	PATHOPHYS-1	Cardiology	7
	CAD—Myocardial Infarction	UCV-2	ER	Cardiology	2
	CAD—Prinzmetal's Angina	MC	ER	Cardiology	2
	CAD—Unstable Angina	MC	ER	Cardiology	3
	Caffeine Intoxication	UCV-1	PHARM	Psychopharmacology	75
	Campylobacter Enteritis	UCV-1	MICRO-1	Infectious Disease	68
	Candida Esophagitis	MC	IM-1	Gastroenterology	100
	Candida Esophagitis	UCV-1	PATHOPHYS-1	Gastroenterology	79
	Candidiasis	UCV-1	MICRO-1	Infectious Disease	69
	Cannabis Intoxication	UCV-1	PHARM	Psychopharmacology	76
	Cannabis Intoxication	UCV-2	PSYCH	Psychopharmacology	18
	Captopril Side Effects	UCV-1	PHARM	Cardiology	3
	Caput Succedaneum	UCV-1	ANAT	Neonatology	43
	Carbamazepine Side Effects	UCV-1	PHARM	Neurology	64
	Carbamazepine Toxicity	MC	NEURO	Neurology	235
	Carbon Dioxide Narcosis	UCV-1	PATHOPHYS-3	Toxicology	97
	Carbon Monoxide Poisoning	UCV-1	BIOCHEM	Pulmonary	95
	Carbon Monoxide Poisoning	UCV-2	ER	Toxicology	47
	Carcinoid Syndrome	MC	IM-1	Gastroenterology	101
	Carcinoid Syndrome	UCV-1	BIOCHEM	Gastroenterology	37
	Cardiac Tamponade	UCV-1	ANAT	Cardiology	3
	Cardiac Tamponade	UCV-1	PATHOPHYS-1	Cardiology	8
	Cardiac Tamponade	UCV-2	ER	Cardiology	3
	Cardiac Transplant	UCV-1	PATHOPHYS-1	Cardiology	9
	Cat-Scratch Disease	UCV-1	MICRO-1	Infectious Disease	70
	Cauda Equina Syndrome	MC	NEURO	Neurology	236
	Cauda Equina Syndrome	UCV-1	PATHOPHYS-3	Neurology	4
	Caustic Ingestion	MC	ER	Toxicology	66
	Cavernous Sinus Thrombosis	MC	NEURO	Neurology	237
	Cavernous Sinus Thrombosis	UCV-1	ANAT	Neurology	55
	Cecal Carcinoma	UCV-1	PATHOPHYS-2	General Surgery	4
	Celiac Disease	MC	IM-1	Gastroenterology	102
	Celiac Disease	UCV-1	PATHOPHYS-1	Gastroenterology	80
	Cellulitis	MC	IM-2	Dermatology	133

Case Name	SER	BOOK	SubSpecialty	Case Number
Cellulitis	UCV-1	MICRO-1	Dermatology	6
Cerebellopontine Angle Compression	MC	NEURO	Neurology	238
Cerebral Aneurysm	MC	NEURO	Neurology	239
Cerebral Aneurysm	UCV-1	PATHOPHYS-3	Neurology	5
Cerebral Palsy	UCV-2	NEURO	Neurology	5
Cervical Carcinoma	UCV-2	OB/GYN	Gynecology	4
Cervical Carcinoma (In Situ)	UCV-1	PATHOPHYS-3	Gynecology	45
Cervical Polyps	MC	OB/GYN	Gynecology	278
Cervicitis	MC	OB/GYN	Gynecology	279
Chagas' Disease	MC	IM-2	Infectious Disease	163
Chagas' Disease	UCV-1	MICRO-1	Infectious Disease	71
Chalazion	MC	ER	ENT/Ophthalmology	38
Chancroid	UCV-2	OB/GYN	Gynecology	5
Chédiak–Higashi Syndrome	MC	IM-2	Genetics	154
Chédiak–Higashi Syndrome	UCV-1	MICRO-1	Genetics	45
Child Abuse—Physical	UCV-2	PED	Psychiatry—Child	53
Child Abuse—Sexual	UCV-2	PSYCH	Child	13
Child Abuse—Shaken Baby Syndrome	UCV-1	BEHAV-SC	Child Psychiatry	34
Chlamydia Pneumonia	MC	IM-2	Infectious Disease	164
Chlamydia Pneumonia	UCV-1	MICRO-1	Infectious Disease	72
Chlamydia trachomatis	UCV-1	MICRO-1	Infectious Disease	73
Chloramphenicol Side Effects	UCV-1	PHARM	Infectious Disease	46
Chloroquine Toxicity	UCV-1	PHARM	Infectious Disease	47
Choanal Atresia	UCV-1	ANAT	ENT/Ophthalmology	10
Choking	UCV-1	ANAT	ENT/Ophthalmology	11
Cholangiocarcinoma	MC	SURG	General Surgery	343
Choledocholithiasis	MC	SURG	General Surgery	344
Cholelithiasis	MC	SURG	General Surgery	345
Cholera	MC	ER	Infectious Disease	57
Cholera	UCV-1	MICRO-1	Infectious Disease	74
Cholestatic Jaundice of Pregnancy	UCV-2	OB/GYN	Obstetrics	37
Chorioamnionitis	UCV-1	MICRO-2	Obstetrics	107
Chorioamnionitis	UCV-2	OB/GYN	Obstetrics	38
Choriocarcinoma	UCV-1	PATHOPHYS-3	Gynecology	46
Choriocarcinoma	UCV-2	OB/GYN	Gynecology	6
Chronic Atrophic Gastritis	MC	IM-1	Gastroenterology	103
Chronic Atrophic Gastritis	UCV-1	PATHOPHYS-1	Gastroenterology	81
Chronic Granulomatous Disease	MC	PED	Immunology	328

Case Name	SER	BOOK	SubSpecialty	Case Number
Chronic Granulomatous Disease	UCV-1	MICRO-2	Immunology	2
Chronic Lymphocytic Leukemia (CLL)	UCV-1	PATHOPHYS-2	Hematology/Oncology	19
Chronic Lymphocytic Leukemia (CLL)	UCV-2	IM-1	Hematology/Oncology	45
Chronic Myelogenous Leukemia (CML)	UCV-1	PATHOPHYS-2	Hematology/Oncology	20
Chronic Myelogenous Leukemia (CML)	UCV-2	IM-1	Hematology/Oncology	46
Chronic Pancreatitis	UCV-1	PATHOPHYS-1	Gastroenterology	82
Chronic Pancreatitis	UCV-2	IM-1	Gastroenterology	29
Churg–Strauss Syndrome	MC	IM-2	Pulmonary	209
Churg–Strauss Syndrome	UCV-1	PATHOPHYS-2	Pulmonary	79
Cimetidine Side Effects	UCV-1	PHARM	Gastroenterology	26
Cisplatin Side Effects	UCV-1	PHARM	Hematology/Oncology	35
Clavicle Fracture	UCV-1	ANAT	Orthopedics	78
Cleft Lip/Palate	MC	PED	General Surgery	314
Clonidine Toxicity	MC	ER	Cardiology	4
Clozapine Toxicity	UCV-1	PHARM	Psychopharmacology	77
Clubfoot	MC	PED	General Surgery	315
Cluster Headache	UCV-2	NEURO	Neurology	6
CMV—Congenital	MC	PED	Infectious Disease	323
CMV—Congenital	UCV-1	MICRO-1	Infectious Disease	75
CMV Pneumonitis	UCV-1	MICRO-1	Infectious Disease	76
CMV Retinitis	UCV-1	MICRO-1	Infectious Disease	77
CMV Retinitis	UCV-2	IM-2	Infectious Disease	15
Coarctation of the Aorta	UCV-1	ANAT	Cardiology	4
Coarctation of the Aorta	UCV-2	SURG	Cardiology	2
Cocaine Abuse	UCV-1	PHARM	Psychopharmacology	78
Cocaine Abuse	UCV-2	PSYCH	Psychopharmacology	19
Cocaine Withdrawal	UCV-1	PHARM	Psychopharmacology	79
Coccidioidomycosis	UCV-1	MICRO-1	Infectious Disease	78
Coccidioidomycosis	UCV-2	IM-2	Infectious Disease	16
Colonic Polyps	MC	SURG	Gastroenterology	340
Colonic Polyps	UCV-1	PATHOPHYS-1	Gastroenterology	83
Colorectal Cancer	UCV-2	SURG	General Surgery	21
Colorado Tick Fever	UCV-1	MICRO-1	Infectious Disease	79
Common Cold (Viral Respiratory Infection)	UCV-1	MICRO-1	ENT/Ophthalmology	20
Common Peroneal Nerve Damage	UCV-1	ANAT	Neurology	56
Conduct Disorder	UCV-1	BEHAV-SC	Child Psychiatry	35
Conduct Disorder	UCV-2	PSYCH	Child	14
Congenital Adrenal Hyperplasia	UCV-1	BIOCHEM	Endocrinology	6

Case Name	SER	BOOK	SubSpecialty	Case Number
Congenital Adrenal Hyperplasia	UCV-2	PED	Endocrinology	5
Congenital Biliary Atresia	UCV-1	ANAT	Gastroenterology	16
Congenital Diaphragmatic Hernia	UCV-1	ANAT	Neonatology	44
Congenital Diaphragmatic Hernia	UCV-2	PED	Neonatology	38
Congenital Prolonged QT Syndrome	MC	PED	Cardiology	296
Congestive Heart Failure	UCV-1	PATHOPHYS-1	Cardiology	10
Congestive Heart Failure	UCV-2	IM-1	Cardiology	4
Constrictive Pericarditis	MC	IM-1	Cardiology	76
Constrictive Pericarditis	UCV-1	PATHOPHYS-1	Cardiology	11
Contact Dermatitis	UCV-1	PATHOPHYS-1	Dermatology	32
Contact Dermatitis	UCV-2	IM-2	Dermatology	4
Conus Medullaris Lesion	MC	NEURO	Neurology	240
Conversion Disorder	UCV-1	BEHAV-SC	Somatoform Disorders	89
Conversion Disorder	UCV-2	PSYCH	SOMATOFORM DISORDERS	51
COPD—Chronic Bronchitis	UCV-2	IM-2	Pulmonary	45
COPD—Chronic Bronchitis	UCV-1	PATHOPHYS-2	Pulmonary	80
COPD—Emphysema	UCV-2	IM-2	Pulmonary	46
COPD—Emphysema	UCV-1	PATHOPHYS-2	Pulmonary	81
Cor Pulmonale	UCV-1	PATHOPHYS-1	Cardiology	12
Cor Pulmonale	UCV-2	IM-1	Cardiology	5
Cord Compression—Extradural	MC	NEURO	Neurology	241
Cord Compression—Intradural	MC	NEURO	Neurology	242
Cord Compression due to Metastasis	UCV-2	ER	Neurology	33
Corneal Abrasion	MC	ER	ENT/Ophthalmology	39
COX-II Inhibitors	UCV-1	PHARM	Orthopedics	71
Coxsackievirus Infections	MC	IM-2	Infectious Disease	165
Craniopharyngioma	UCV-1	PATHOPHYS-3	Neurology	6
Craniopharyngioma	UCV-2	NEURO	Neurology	7
Creutzfeldt–Jakob Disease	UCV-1	PATHOPHYS-3	Neurology	7
Creutzfeldt–Jakob Disease	UCV-2	NEURO	Neurology	8
Cribriform Plate Fracture	UCV-1	PATHOPHYS-1	ENT/Ophthalmology	64
Crigler–Najjar Syndrome	MC	PED	Gastroenterology	311
Crigler–Najjar Syndrome	UCV-1	BIOCHEM	Gastroenterology	38
Crohn's Disease	UCV-1	PATHOPHYS-1	Gastroenterology	84
Crohn's Disease	UCV-2	IM-1	Gastroenterology	30
Croup	UCV-1	MICRO-1	Infectious Disease	80
Croup	UCV-2	PED	Infectious Disease	28
Cryptosporidiosis	MC	IM-2	Infectious Disease	166

Case Name	SER	BOOK	SubSpecialty	Case Number
Delirium	UCV-2	PSYCH	Neurology	1
Delirium—Inhalant Abuse	UCV-1	BEHAV-SC	Neurology	3
Delirium—Medical Cause	UCV-1	BEHAV-SC	Neurology	4
Delirium Tremens	UCV-2	PSYCH	Psychopharmacology	20
Delusional Disorder	UCV-1	BEHAV-SC	Psychotic Disorders	78
Delusional Disorder	UCV-2	PSYCH	Psychotic Disorders	48
Dementia—Alzheimer's	UCV-2	PSYCH	Neurology	2
Dementia—Alzheimer's	UCV-1	BEHAV-SC	Neurology	5
Dementia—Vascular	UCV-2	NEURO	Neurology	17
Dementia—Vascular	UCV-1	BEHAV-SC	Neurology	6
Denial	UCV-1	BEHAV-SC	Defense Mechanism	14
Dependent Personality Disorder	UCV-1	BEHAV-SC	Personality Disorders	69
Depression—Elderly	UCV-1	BEHAV-SC	Mood Disorders	53
Depression—Suicidal	UCV-2	ER	Psychiatry-Mood Disorders	44
Depression—Suicidal	UCV-1	BEHAV-SC	Mood Disorders	54
Depression due to a Medical Condition	UCV-2	PSYCH	Mood Disorders	41
Depressive Episode—Major	UCV-2	PSYCH	Mood Disorders	42
Depressive Episode—Major	UCV-1	BEHAV-SC	Mood Disorders	55
Dermatitis Herpetiformis	UCV-1	PATHOPHYS-1	Dermatology	33
Dermatitis Herpetiformis	UCV-2	IM-2	Dermatology	5
Dermatomyositis	UCV-1	PATHOPHYS-3	Rheumatology	81
Dermatomyositis	UCV-2	IM-2	Rheumatology	51
Desmoid Tumor	UCV-1	PATHOPHYS-3	Gynecology	47
Devaluation	UCV-1	BEHAV-SC	Defense Mechanism	15
Diabetes in Pregnancy	UCV-2	OB/GYN	Obstetrics	39
Diabetes Insipidus	UCV-1	BIOCHEM	Endocrinology	7
Diabetes Mellitus Type I (Juvenile Onset)	UCV-1	PATHOPHYS-1	Endocrinology	51
Diabetes Mellitus Type I (Juvenile Onset)	UCV-2	IM-1	Endocrinology	18
Diabetes Mellitus Type II (Adult Onset)	MC	IM-1	Endocrinology	88
Diabetes Mellitus Type II (Adult Onset)	UCV-1	PATHOPHYS-1	Endocrinology	52
Diabetic Ketoacidosis	UCV-1	BIOCHEM	Endocrinology	8
Diabetic Ketoacidosis	UCV-2	IM-1	Endocrinology	19
Diabetic Nephropathy	MC	IM-2	Nephrology/Urology	198
Diabetic Nephropathy	UCV-1	PATHOPHYS-2	Nephrology/Urology	55
Diagnosis of Pregnancy	UCV-2	OB/GYN	Obstetrics	40
Diaper Rash	MC	PED	Dermatology	298
Didanosine Toxicity	UCV-1	PHARM	Toxicology	98
Diethylstilbestrol (DES) Exposure	UCV-1	PHARM	Endocrinology	16

Case Name	SER	BOOK	SubSpecialty	Case Number
DiGeorge's Syndrome	MC	PED	Immunology	329
DiGeorge's Syndrome (Thymic Aplasia)	UCV-1	ANAT	Immunology	42
Digitalis Intoxication	UCV-1	PHARM	Cardiology	4
Dilated Cardiomyopathy	UCV-1	PATHOPHYS-1	Cardiology	13
Dilated Cardiomyopathy	UCV-2	IM-1	Cardiology	6
Diphtheria	MC	PED	Infectious Disease	324
Diphtheria	UCV-1	MICRO-1	Infectious Disease	82
Disclosure of Teen Pregnancy	UCV-2	PSYCH	Ethics	30
Discoid Lupus Erythematosus	MC	IM-2	Dermatology	134
Displacement	UCV-1	BEHAV-SC	Defense Mechanism	16
Disseminated Gonorrhea	UCV-2	OB/GYN	Gynecology	7
Disseminated Intravascular Coagulation (DIC)	UCV-1	PATHOPHYS-2	Hematology/Oncology	22
Disseminated Intravascular Coagulation (DIC)	UCV-2	IM-1	Hematology/Oncology	47
Dissociative Amnesia	UCV-1	BEHAV-SC	Dissociative Identity Disorder	41
Dissociative Disorder (Depersonalization)	UCV-1	BEHAV-SC	Dissociative Identity Disorder	42
Dissociative Fugue	UCV-1	BEHAV-SC	Dissociative Identity Disorder	43
Dissociative Identity Disorder	UCV-1	BEHAV-SC	Dissociative Identity Disorder	44
Diverticulitis	UCV-1	PATHOPHYS-1	Gastroenterology	85
Diverticulitis	UCV-2	SURG	Gastroenterology	11
Diverticulosis	UCV-1	PATHOPHYS-1	Gastroenterology	86
Diverticulosis	UCV-2	IM-1	Gastroenterology	31
Domestic Violence	UCV-2	ER	Psychiatry—Ethics	43
Down's Syndrome	MC	PED	Genetics	317
Down's Syndrome	UCV-1	PATHOPHYS-2	Genetics	11
Doxorubicin Cardiotoxicity	UCV-1	PHARM	Hematology/Oncology	37
Drug Induced Lupus	UCV-1	PHARM	Rheumatology	91
Drug Resistance	UCV-1	PHARM	Infectious Disease	48
Drug-Induced Lupus	MC	IM-2	Rheumatology	220
Drug-Induced Neutropenia	MC	IM-1	Hematology/Oncology	120
Dubin–Johnson Syndrome	UCV-1	BIOCHEM	Gastroenterology	39
Duchenne's Muscular Dystrophy	UCV-1	BIOCHEM	Neurology	85
Duchenne's Muscular Dystrophy	UCV-2	PED	Neurology	49
Dumping Syndrome	UCV-1	ANAT	Gastroenterology	17
Duodenal Atresia	UCV-1	ANAT	Neonatology	45
Duodenal Atresia	UCV-2	PED	Neonatology	39
Dysbetalipoproteinemia	UCV-1	PATHOPHYS-2	Hematology/Oncology	23

	Case Name	SER	BOOK	SubSpecialty	Case Number
	Dysfunctional Uterine Bleeding	UCV-2	OB/GYN	Gynecology	8
	Dysmenorrhea	MC	OB/GYN	Gynecology	280
	Dysmenorrhea	UCV-1	PATHOPHYS-3	Gynecology	48
	Dysplastic Nevi	MC	IM-2	Dermatology	135
	Dysplastic Nevus Syndrome	UCV-1	PATHOPHYS-1	Dermatology	34
	Dysthymic Disorder	UCV-1	BEHAV-SC	Mood Disorders	56
	Dysthymic Disorder	UCV-2	PSYCH	Mood Disorders	43
E	Eaton–Lambert Syndrome	MC	NEURO	Neurology	243
	Echinococcosis	MC	IM-2	Infectious Disease	167
	Echinococcosis	UCV-1	MICRO-1	Infectious Disease	83
	Ectopic Pregnancy	UCV-1	PATHOPHYS-3	Obstetrics	63
	Ectopic Pregnancy	UCV-2	OB/GYN	Obstetrics	41
	Ectopic Pregnancy—Ruptured	UCV-1	ANAT	Obstetrics	74
	Ehlers–Danlos Syndrome	MC	PED	Genetics	318
	Ehlers–Danlos Syndrome	UCV-1	BIOCHEM	Genetics	47
	Ehrlichiosis	MC	IM-2	Infectious Disease	168
	Ehrlichiosis	UCV-1	MICRO-1	Infectious Disease	84
	Eisenmenger's Complex	MC	PED	Cardiology	297
	Eisenmenger's Complex	UCV-1	PATHOPHYS-1	Cardiology	14
	Elbow—Lateral Epicondylitis	UCV-1	ANAT	Orthopedics	79
	Elbow—Median Nerve Palsy (Noncarpal)	UCV-1	ANAT	Orthopedics	80
	Elbow—Radial Head Subluxation	UCV-1	ANAT	Orthopedics	81
	Electric Shock	UCV-2	ER	General Surgery	16
	Electromechanical Dissociation	MC	ER	Cardiology	7
	Endemic Typhus	UCV-1	MICRO-1	Infectious Disease	85
	Endometrial Carcinoma	UCV-1	PATHOPHYS-3	Gynecology	49
	Endometrial Carcinoma	UCV-2	OB/GYN	Gynecology	9
	Endometriosis	UCV-1	PATHOPHYS-3	Gynecology	50
	Endometriosis	UCV-2	OB/GYN	Gynecology	10
	Enuresis	UCV-1	BEHAV-SC	Child Psychiatry	36
	Epidemic Typhus	MC	IM-2	Infectious Disease	169
	Epidemic Typhus	UCV-1	MICRO-1	Infectious Disease	86
	Epidemic Typhus	UCV-2	IM-2	Infectious Disease	17
	Epidermal Inclusion Cyst	MC	SURG	Dermatology	336
	Epididymitis	MC	SURG	Nephrology/Urology	365
	Epididymitis	UCV-1	MICRO-2	Nephrology/Urology	81
	Epidural Hematoma	UCV-1	PATHOPHYS-3	Neurology	10
	Epidural Hematoma	UCV-2	SURG	Neurology	40

	Case Name	SER	BOOK	SubSpecialty	Case Number
	Epiglottitis	UCV-1	MICRO-1	Infectious Disease	87
	Epiglottitis	UCV-2	ER	Infectious Disease	25
	Epiphyseal Separation with Ulnar Nerve Palsy	UCV-1	ANAT	Neurology	58
	Epispadias	MC	SURG	General Surgery	348
	Erb's Palsy	UCV-1	ANAT	Neurology	59
	Erysipelas	MC	IM-2	Dermatology	136
	Erysipelas	UCV-1	MICRO-1	Dermatology	7
	Erysipeloid	MC	IM-2	Dermatology	137
	Erysipeloid	UCV-1	MICRO-1	Dermatology	8
	Erythema Infectiosum	MC	PED	Dermatology	299
	Erythema Infectiosum	UCV-1	MICRO-1	Dermatology	9
	Erythema Multiforme	MC	ER	Dermatology	18
	Erythema Multiforme	UCV-1	PATHOPHYS-1	Dermatology	35
	Erythema Nodosum	UCV-2	IM-2	Dermatology	6
	Erythroblastosis Fetalis	UCV-1	PATHOPHYS-2	Neonatology	46
	Erythroblastosis Fetalis	UCV-2	PED	Neonatology	40
	Erythroderma	MC	IM-2	Dermatology	138
	Esophageal Carcinoma	UCV-1	PATHOPHYS-2	General Surgery	5
	Esophageal Carcinoma	UCV-2	SURG	General Surgery	22
	Esophageal Spasm	MC	ER	Gastroenterology	46
	Esophageal Spasm	UCV-1	PATHOPHYS-1	Gastroenterology	87
	Esophageal Variceal Bleeding	UCV-1	PATHOPHYS-1	Gastroenterology	88
	Essential Thrombocythemia	MC	IM-1	Hematology/Oncology	121
	Ethylene Glycol Ingestion	MC	ER	Toxicology	68
	Ethylene Glycol Ingestion	UCV-1	PHARM	Toxicology	99
	Ewing's Sarcoma	MC	SURG	Orthopedics	369
	Ewing's Sarcoma	UCV-1	PATHOPHYS-3	Orthopedics	68
	Exhibitionism	UCV-1	BEHAV-SC	Paraphilia	60
F	Fabry's Disease	UCV-1	BIOCHEM	Genetics	48
	Facial Nerve Injury	UCV-1	ANAT	Neurology	60
	Factitious Disorder	UCV-2	PSYCH	Factitious Disorder	36
	Familial Hypercholesterolemia	UCV-1	BIOCHEM	Genetics	49
	Familial Hypertriglyceridemia	UCV-1	BIOCHEM	Genetics	50
	Fanconi's Anemia	UCV-1	BIOCHEM	Genetics	51
	Fat Embolism	MC	ER	Pulmonary	63
	Fat Embolism	UCV-1	PATHOPHYS-2	Pulmonary	82
	Felty's Syndrome	MC	IM-2	Rheumatology	221

	Case Name	SER	BOOK	SubSpecialty	Case Number
	Femoral Hematoma	UCV-1	ANAT	Cardiology	5
	Femoral Hernia—Strangulated	UCV-1	ANAT	General Surgery	25
	Femoral Nerve Palsy	UCV-1	ANAT	Neurology	61
	Fetal Alcohol Syndrome	MC	NEURO	Neurology	244
	Fetal Alcohol Syndrome	UCV-1	PHARM	Neurology	65
	Fetal Neglect	UCV-2	PSYCH	Ethics	31
	Fetishism	UCV-1	BEHAV-SC	Paraphilia	61
	Fitz-Hugh–Curtis Syndrome	UCV-1	MICRO-1	Gastroenterology	27
	Fixation	UCV-1	BEHAV-SC	Defense Mechanism	17
	Flail Chest	MC	ER	Pulmonary	64
	Fluoroquinolone Side Effects	UCV-1	PHARM	Infectious Disease	49
	Forearm—Galeazzi's Fracture	MC	SURG	Orthopedics	370
	Forearm—Monteggia's Fracture	MC	SURG	Orthopedics	371
	Forearm—Monteggia's Fracture	UCV-1	ANAT	Orthopedics	82
	Foreign Body—Ear	MC	ER	ENT/Ophthalmology	40
	Foreign Body—Rectum	MC	ER	Gastroenterology	47
	Foreign Body—Trachea	MC	ER	ENT/Ophthalmology	41
	Foreign Body Ingestion	MC	ER	Gastroenterology	45
	Fragile X Syndrome	UCV-1	BIOCHEM	Genetics	52
	Friedreich's Ataxia	UCV-1	PATHOPHYS-3	Neurology	11
	Friedreich's Ataxia	UCV-2	NEURO	Neurology	18
	Frost Bite	MC	ER	General Surgery	53
	Frotteurism	UCV-1	BEHAV-SC	Paraphilia	62
	Fulminant Hepatic Failure	MC	ER	Gastroenterology	48
	Furuncle	MC	IM-2	Dermatology	139
	Furuncle	UCV-1	PATHOPHYS-1	Dermatology	36
G	Galactosemia	UCV-1	BIOCHEM	Genetics	53
	Gallstone Ileus	UCV-2	SURG	General Surgery	24
	Gartner's Duct Cyst	UCV-1	ANAT	Gynecology	39
	Gas Gangrene—Traumatic	UCV-1	MICRO-1	Infectious Disease	88
	Gastric Carcinoma	UCV-1	PATHOPHYS-2	General Surgery	6
	Gastric Carcinoma	UCV-2	SURG	General Surgery	25
	Gastric Leiomyoma	UCV-1	PATHOPHYS-2	General Surgery	7
	Gastroenteritis	MC	ER	Gastroenterology	49
	Gastroenteritis	UCV-2	PED	Gastroenterology	7
	Gastroenteritis—*Staphylococcus aureus*	UCV-1	MICRO-1	Gastroenterology	28
	Gastroesophageal Reflux Disease (GERD)	UCV-1	PATHOPHYS-1	Gastroenterology	89

Case Name	SER	BOOK	SubSpecialty	Case Number
Gastroesophageal Reflux Disease (GERD)	UCV-2	IM-1	Gastroenterology	32
Gastrointestinal Bleeding—Lower	UCV-2	SURG	General Surgery	26
Gastrointestinal Bleeding—Upper	UCV-2	SURG	General Surgery	27
Gaucher's Disease	MC	PED	Genetics	319
Gaucher's Disease	UCV-1	BIOCHEM	Genetics	54
Gender Identity Disorder	UCV-1	BEHAV-SC	Gender Identity Disorder	49
Gender Identity Disorder	UCV-2	PSYCH	Gender Identity Disorder	38
Generalized Anxiety Disorder	UCV-1	BEHAV-SC	Anxiety Disorders	27
Generalized Anxiety Disorder	UCV-2	PSYCH	Anxiety Disorders	6
Gentamicin Side Effects	MC	IM-2	Infectious Disease	170
Gentamicin Side Effects	UCV-1	PHARM	Infectious Disease	50
Gerstmann–Sträussler–Scheinker Syndrome	MC	NEURO	Neurology	245
Giardiasis	MC	IM-2	Infectious Disease	171
Giardiasis	UCV-1	MICRO-1	Infectious Disease	89
Gilbert's Disease	MC	IM-1	Gastroenterology	104
Gilbert's Disease	UCV-1	BIOCHEM	Gastroenterology	40
Glioblastoma Multiforme	UCV-1	PATHOPHYS-3	Neurology	12
Glioblastoma Multiforme	UCV-2	NEURO	Neurology	19
Glucagonoma	UCV-1	BIOCHEM	Endocrinology	9
Glucagonoma	UCV-2	IM-1	Endocrinology	20
Glucose-6-Phosphate Dehydrogenase (G6PD) Deficiency	MC	IM-1	Hematology/Oncology	122
Glucose-6-Phosphate Dehydrogenase (G6PD) Deficiency	UCV-1	BIOCHEM	Hematology/Oncology	78
Glycogen Storage Diseases	MC	PED	Genetics	320
Gonococcal Ophthalmia Neonatorum	UCV-1	MICRO-1	Infectious Disease	90
Gonorrhea	UCV-1	MICRO-1	Infectious Disease	91
Gonorrhea	UCV-2	IM-2	Infectious Disease	18
Goodpasture's Syndrome	MC	IM-2	Nephrology/Urology	199
Goodpasture's Syndrome	UCV-1	PATHOPHYS-2	Nephrology/Urology	56
Gout	UCV-1	BIOCHEM	Rheumatology	95
Gout	UCV-2	IM-2	Rheumatology	52
Graft-Versus-Host Disease	UCV-1	MICRO-1	Hematology/Oncology	48
Granuloma Inguinale	MC	IM-2	Infectious Disease	172
Granuloma Inguinale	UCV-1	MICRO-1	Infectious Disease	92
Grief—Normal	UCV-1	BEHAV-SC	Mood Disorders	57
Grief—Pathologic	UCV-1	BEHAV-SC	Mood Disorders	58

	Case Name	SER	BOOK	SubSpecialty	Case Number
	Guillain–Barré Syndrome	UCV-1	PATHOPHYS-3	Neurology	13
	Guillain–Barré Syndrome	UCV-2	NEURO	Neurology	20
H	*H influenzae* in a COPD Patient	UCV-1	MICRO-1	Infectious Disease	93
	Hairy Cell Leukemia	MC	IM-1	Hematology/Oncology	123
	Hairy Cell Leukemia	UCV-1	PATHOPHYS-2	Hematology/Oncology	24
	Hand—Boxer's Fracture	UCV-1	ANAT	Orthopedics	83
	Hand—Dupuytren's Contracture	UCV-1	PATHOPHYS-3	Orthopedics	69
	Hand—Dupuytren's Contracture	UCV-2	SURG	Orthopedics	41
	Hantavirus Pulmonary Syndrome	UCV-1	MICRO-1	Infectious Disease	94
	Hashimoto's Thyroiditis	UCV-1	PATHOPHYS-1	Endocrinology	53
	Hashimoto's Thyroiditis	UCV-2	IM-1	Endocrinology	21
	Heart Block	MC	ER	Cardiology	8
	Heat Stroke	MC	ER	Cardiology	9
	Heavy Metals Toxicity	MC	ER	Toxicology	69
	HELLP Syndrome	MC	OB/GYN	Obstetrics	291
	Hemangioma	MC	SURG	General Surgery	349
	Hemiballismus	UCV-1	PATHOPHYS-3	Neurology	14
	Hemochromatosis	UCV-1	PATHOPHYS-1	Gastroenterology	90
	Hemochromatosis	UCV-2	IM-1	Gastroenterology	33
	Hemolytic-Uremic Syndrome (HUS)	MC	IM-1	Hematology/Oncology	124
	Hemolytic-Uremic Syndrome (HUS)	UCV-1	MICRO-1	Hematology/Oncology	49
	Hemophilia	UCV-2	PED	Hematology/Oncology	18
	Hemophilia, Type A	UCV-1	BIOCHEM	Hematology/Oncology	79
	Hemorrhagic Fever—Crimean-Congo	UCV-1	MICRO-1	Infectious Disease	95
	Hemorrhagic Fever—Dengue	UCV-1	MICRO-1	Infectious Disease	96
	Hemorrhagic Fever—Ebola Virus	UCV-1	MICRO-1	Infectious Disease	97
	Hemorrhagic Fever Renal Syndrome	UCV-1	MICRO-1	Infectious Disease	98
	Hemorrhagic Gastritis—Drug-Induced	MC	ER	Gastroenterology	50
	Hemorrhagic Gastritis—Drug-Induced	UCV-1	PHARM	Gastroenterology	27
	Hemorrhoids—External	MC	SURG	General Surgery	350
	Hemorrhoids—Internal	MC	SURG	General Surgery	351
	Hemorrhoids—Internal-External	UCV-2	SURG	General Surgery	28
	Hemorrhoids—Thrombosed External	UCV-1	ANAT	General Surgery	26
	Henoch–Schönlein Purpura	UCV-1	PATHOPHYS-2	Hematology/Oncology	25
	Henoch–Schönlein Purpura	UCV-2	PED	Hematology/Oncology	19
	Heparin Overdose	UCV-1	PHARM	Hematology/Oncology	38
	Heparin Toxicity	MC	ER	Hematology/Oncology	55
	Hepatic Cirrhosis	UCV-1	PATHOPHYS-1	Gastroenterology	91

Case Name	SER	BOOK	SubSpecialty	Case Number
Hepatic Cirrhosis	UCV-2	IM-1	Gastroenterology	34
Hepatic Encephalopathy	MC	ER	Gastroenterology	51
Hepatic Encephalopathy	UCV-1	PATHOPHYS-1	Gastroenterology	92
Hepatitis—Alcoholic	UCV-1	PATHOPHYS-1	Gastroenterology	93
Hepatitis—Chronic Active	MC	IM-1	Gastroenterology	105
Hepatitis—Halothane	UCV-1	PHARM	Gastroenterology	28
Hepatitis—INH	UCV-1	PHARM	Gastroenterology	29
Hepatitis A	UCV-1	MICRO-1	Gastroenterology	29
Hepatitis A	UCV-2	IM-1	Gastroenterology	35
Hepatitis B—Acute	UCV-1	MICRO-1	Gastroenterology	30
Hepatitis C—Chronic Active	UCV-1	MICRO-1	Gastroenterology	31
Hepatitis, Chronic (Alcoholic)	UCV-2	IM-1	Gastroenterology	36
Hepatocellular Carcinoma	MC	IM-1	Gastroenterology	106
Hepatocellular Carcinoma	UCV-1	PATHOPHYS-1	Gastroenterology	94
Hepatorenal Syndrome	MC	IM-1	Gastroenterology	107
Hepatorenal Syndrome	UCV-1	PATHOPHYS-1	Gastroenterology	95
Hereditary Angioedema	MC	PED	Immunology	330
Hereditary Angioedema	UCV-1	MICRO-2	Immunology	3
Hereditary Fructose Intolerance	UCV-1	BIOCHEM	Genetics	55
Hereditary Spherocytosis	UCV-1	BIOCHEM	Hematology/Oncology	80
Hereditary Spherocytosis	UCV-2	IM-1	Hematology/Oncology	48
Heroin Overdose	UCV-1	PHARM	Psychopharmacology	80
Heroin Overdose	UCV-2	ER	Psychopharmacology	40
Herpangina	MC	IM-2	Infectious Disease	173
Herpangina	UCV-1	MICRO-1	Infectious Disease	99
Herpes Genitalis	UCV-1	MICRO-1	Infectious Disease	100
Herpes Genitalis	UCV-2	IM-2	Infectious Disease	19
Herpes Labialis	MC	IM-2	Infectious Disease	174
Herpes Simplex Encephalitis	UCV-1	MICRO-2	Neurology	89
Herpes Simplex Encephalitis	UCV-2	NEURO	Neurology	21
Herpes Zoster (Shingles)	UCV-1	MICRO-1	Infectious Disease	101
Herpes Zoster (Shingles)	UCV-2	IM-2	Infectious Disease	20
Herpes Zoster Ophthalmicus	MC	ER	ENT/Ophthalmology	31
Herpes Zoster Ophthalmicus	UCV-1	MICRO-1	ENT/Ophthalmology	21
Hiatal Hernia	MC	SURG	Gastroenterology	341
Hiatal Hernia	UCV-1	ANAT	Gastroenterology	18
High-Altitude Sickness	UCV-1	PATHOPHYS-1	Cardiology	15
Hip—Avascular Necrosis of the Femoral He	UCV-1	PATHOPHYS-3	Orthopedics	70

Case Name	SER	BOOK	SubSpecialty	Case Number
Hip—Legg–Calve–Perthes Disease	UCV-1	ANAT	Orthopedics	84
Hip—Slipped Capital Femoral Epiphysis	MC	SURG	Orthopedics	372
Hip—Slipped Capital Femoral Epiphysis	UCV-1	PATHOPHYS-3	Orthopedics	71
Hip—Trendelenburg Gait	UCV-1	ANAT	Orthopedics	85
Hip Dislocation—Congenital	UCV-1	ANAT	Orthopedics	86
Hip Dislocation—Congenital	UCV-2	PED	Orthopedics	51
Hip Dislocation—Traumatic	UCV-2	SURG	Orthopedics	42
Hip Dislocation—Traumatic	UCV-1	ANAT	Orthopedics	87
Hip Fracture	UCV-1	ANAT	Orthopedics	88
Hip Fracture	UCV-2	SURG	Orthopedics	43
Hirschsprung's Disease	MC	PED	Gastroenterology	312
Hirschsprung's Disease	UCV-1	ANAT	Gastroenterology	19
Hirsutism—Idiopathic	MC	OB/GYN	Endocrinology	270
Hirsutism—Idiopathic	UCV-1	BIOCHEM	Endocrinology	10
Histiocytosis X—Eosinophilic Granuloma	UCV-1	PATHOPHYS-2	Hematology/Oncology	26
Histiocytosis X—Hand–Schüller–Christian Disease	UCV-1	PATHOPHYS-2	Hematology/Oncology	27
Histiocytosis X—Letterer–Siwe Disease	UCV-1	PATHOPHYS-2	Hematology/Oncology	28
Histoplasmosis	UCV-1	MICRO-2	Infectious Disease	7
Histoplasmosis	UCV-2	IM-2	Infectious Disease	21
Histrionic Personality Disorder	UCV-1	BEHAV-SC	Personality Disorders	70
HIV Transmission in Pregnancy	MC	OB/GYN	Obstetrics	292
HIV Transmission in Pregnancy	UCV-1	MICRO-2	Obstetrics	108
HIV/AIDS	MC	IM-2	Infectious Disease	175
Hodgkin's Lymphoma	UCV-1	PATHOPHYS-2	Hematology/Oncology	29
Hodgkin's Lymphoma	UCV-2	IM-1	Hematology/Oncology	49
Homocystinuria	UCV-1	BIOCHEM	Genetics	56
Homocystinuria	UCV-2	PED	Genetics	12
Hookworm	UCV-1	MICRO-1	Gastroenterology	32
Horner's Syndrome	UCV-2	NEURO	Neurology	22
HSV Keratitis	UCV-1	MICRO-1	ENT/Ophthalmology	22
Human Bite	MC	IM-2	Infectious Disease	176
Human Papilloma Virus (HPV)—Plantar Warts	MC	IM-2	Dermatology	140
Human Papillomavirus (HPV)	UCV-1	MICRO-2	Gynecology	103
Human Papillomavirus (HPV)	UCV-2	OB/GYN	Gynecology	11
Human Papillomavirus (HPV)—Common Wart	MC	IM-2	Dermatology	141
Human Papillomavirus (HPV)—Common Wart	MC	IM-1	Dermatology	94
Human T-Cell Leukemia Virus Type 1 (HTLV-1)	UCV-1	MICRO-2	Infectious Disease	8

Case Name	SER	BOOK	SubSpecialty	Case Number
Hunter's Disease	UCV-1	BIOCHEM	Genetics	57
Huntington's Chorea	UCV-1	PATHOPHYS-3	Neurology	15
Huntington's Disease	UCV-2	NEURO	Neurology	23
Hurler's Disease	UCV-1	BIOCHEM	Genetics	58
Hyaline Membrane Disease	UCV-1	BIOCHEM	Pulmonary	91
Hyaline Membrane Disease	UCV-2	PED	Neonatology	41
Hydatidiform Mole	UCV-1	PATHOPHYS-3	Gynecology	51
Hydatidiform Mole	UCV-2	OB/GYN	Gynecology	12
Hyperaldosteronism—Primary	UCV-1	BIOCHEM	Endocrinology	11
Hyperaldosteronism—Primary	UCV-2	SURG	Endocrinology	6
Hyperaldosteronism—Secondary	MC	IM-1	Endocrinology	89
Hypercalcemia	UCV-1	BIOCHEM	Endocrinology	12
Hyperemesis Gravidarum	UCV-2	OB/GYN	Obstetrics	42
Hyperkalemia	UCV-2	IM-2	Nephrology/Urology	34
Hyperparathyroidism—Primary	UCV-1	BIOCHEM	Endocrinology	13
Hyperparathyroidism—Primary	UCV-2	IM-1	Endocrinology	22
Hypersensitivity Pneumonitis	MC	IM-2	Pulmonary	210
Hypersensitivity Pneumonitis	UCV-1	PATHOPHYS-2	Pulmonary	83
Hypertension—Essential	MC	IM-1	Cardiology	77
Hypertensive Renal Disease	UCV-1	PATHOPHYS-2	Nephrology/Urology	57
Hyperthyroidism (Graves' Disease)	MC	IM-1	Endocrinology	90
Hyperthyroidism (Graves' Disease)	UCV-1	BIOCHEM	Endocrinology	14
Hyperthyroidism (Solitary Nodule)	MC	SURG	Endocrinology	338
Hyperthyroidism (Solitary Nodule)	UCV-1	PATHOPHYS-1	Endocrinology	54
Hypertrophic Obstructive Cardiomyopathy	UCV-1	PATHOPHYS-1	Cardiology	16
Hypertrophic Obstructive Cardiomyopathy	UCV-2	IM-1	Cardiology	7
Hypertrophic Pyloric Stenosis	UCV-1	ANAT	Neonatology	46
Hypertrophic Pyloric Stenosis	UCV-2	PED	Neonatology	42
Hyperventilation	UCV-1	BIOCHEM	Pulmonary	93
Hypocalcemia from Pancreatitis	UCV-1	BIOCHEM	Endocrinology	15
Hypochondriasis	UCV-1	BEHAV-SC	Somatoform Disorders	90
Hypochondriasis	UCV-2	PSYCH	Somatoform Disorders	52
Hypoglossal Nerve Palsy	UCV-1	ANAT	Neurology	62
Hypokalemia	UCV-1	BIOCHEM	Endocrinology	16
Hypomagnesemia	UCV-1	BIOCHEM	Endocrinology	17
Hyponatremia	UCV-1	BIOCHEM	Endocrinology	18
Hypoparathyroidism	UCV-2	IM-1	Endocrinology	23
Hypoparathyroidism—Iatrogenic	UCV-1	ANAT	Endocrinology	9

	Case Name	SER	BOOK	SubSpecialty	Case Number
	Hypopituitarism	MC	IM-1	Endocrinology	91
	Hypopituitarism	UCV-1	PATHOPHYS-1	Endocrinology	55
	Hypospadias	MC	SURG	General Surgery	352
	Hypothermia	UCV-1	PATHOPHYS-1	Cardiology	17
	Hypothermia	UCV-2	ER	Cardiology	4
	Hypothyroidism—Congenital	UCV-1	PATHOPHYS-1	Endocrinology	56
	Hypothyroidism—Congenital	UCV-2	PED	Endocrinology	6
	Hypothyroidism—Myxedema Coma	MC	ER	Endocrinology	22
	Hypothyroidism—Primary	UCV-1	PATHOPHYS-1	Endocrinology	57
	Hypothyroidism—Primary	UCV-2	IM-1	Endocrinology	24
I	ICU Psychosis	UCV-1	BEHAV-SC	Psychotic Disorders	79
	Identification	UCV-1	BEHAV-SC	Defense Mechanism	18
	Idiopathic Pulmonary Fibrosis (IPF)	UCV-1	PATHOPHYS-2	Pulmonary	84
	Idiopathic Thrombocytopenic Purpura (ITP)	UCV-1	PATHOPHYS-2	Hematology/Oncology	30
	Idiopathic Thrombocytopenic Purpura (ITP)	UCV-2	PED	Hematology/Oncology	20
	IgA Nephropathy (Berger's Disease)	MC	IM-2	Nephrology/Urology	200
	IgA Nephropathy (Berger's Disease)	UCV-1	PATHOPHYS-2	Nephrology/Urology	58
	Impetigo	UCV-1	MICRO-1	Dermatology	10
	Impetigo	UCV-2	PED	Dermatology	4
	Inclusion Conjunctivitis	UCV-1	MICRO-2	Infectious Disease	9
	Infectious Mononucleosis	UCV-1	MICRO-2	Infectious Disease	10
	Infectious Mononucleosis	UCV-2	IM-2	Infectious Disease	22
	Infertility	UCV-2	OB/GYN	Gynecology	13
	Influenza	MC	IM-2	Infectious Disease	177
	Influenza	UCV-1	MICRO-2	Infectious Disease	11
	Inguinal Hernia	UCV-2	SURG	General Surgery	29
	Inguinal Hernia—Direct	UCV-1	ANAT	General Surgery	27
	Inguinal Hernia—Indirect	UCV-1	ANAT	General Surgery	28
	Insulin Overdose	UCV-1	PHARM	Endocrinology	17
	Insulinoma	UCV-1	BIOCHEM	Endocrinology	19
	Insulinoma	UCV-2	IM-1	Endocrinology	25
	Interferon Use	UCV-1	PHARM	Immunology	44
	Internuclear Ophthalmoplegia	UCV-1	PATHOPHYS-3	Neurology	16
	Interstitial Cystitis	MC	IM-2	Nephrology/Urology	201
	Interstitial Lung Disease	MC	IM-2	Pulmonary	211
	Intestinal Malrotation with Volvulus	MC	SURG	General Surgery	353

	Case Name	SER	BOOK	SubSpecialty	Case Number
	Intestinal Obstruction	UCV-2	SURG	General Surgery	30
	Intestinal Obstruction—Acute	UCV-1	PATHOPHYS-2	General Surgery	8
	Intestinal Perforation	MC	SURG	General Surgery	354
	Intra-Abdominal Abscess	UCV-2	SURG	General Surgery	31
	Intrahepatic Cholestasis of Pregnancy	MC	OB/GYN	Obstetrics	293
	Intussusception	UCV-1	PATHOPHYS-2	General Surgery	9
	Intussusception	UCV-2	ER	General Surgery	17
	Ipecac Toxicity	UCV-1	PHARM	Toxicology	100
	Iron Overdose	UCV-1	PHARM	Hematology/Oncology	39
	Irritable Bowel Syndrome	UCV-2	IM-1	Gastroenterology	37
	Isolation of Affect	UCV-1	BEHAV-SC	Defense Mechanism	19
J	Japanese Encephalitis	UCV-1	MICRO-2	Neurology	90
	Jarisch–Herxheimer Reaction	UCV-1	MICRO-2	Infectious Disease	12
	Juvenile Rheumatoid Arthritis	UCV-1	PATHOPHYS-3	Rheumatology	82
	Juvenile Rheumatoid Arthritis	UCV-2	PED	Rheumatology	55
K	Kallmann's Syndrome	UCV-1	BIOCHEM	Endocrinology	20
	Kaposi's Sarcoma	UCV-1	PATHOPHYS-1	Dermatology	37
	Kaposi's Sarcoma	UCV-2	IM-2	Dermatology	7
	Kartagener's Syndrome	MC	IM-2	Genetics	155
	Kartagener's Syndrome	UCV-1	BIOCHEM	Genetics	59
	Kawasaki Syndrome	MC	PED	Dermatology	300
	Kawasaki's Syndrome	UCV-1	PATHOPHYS-1	Dermatology	38
	Ketamine Side Effects	UCV-1	PHARM	Neurology	66
	Ketoconazole Side Effects	UCV-1	PHARM	Infectious Disease	51
	Klatskin Tumor	MC	SURG	General Surgery	355
	Klinefelter's Syndrome	MC	PED	Genetics	321
	Klinefelter's Syndrome	UCV-1	BIOCHEM	Genetics	60
	Klumpke's Palsy	MC	NEURO	Neurology	246
	Klumpke's Palsy	UCV-1	ANAT	Neurology	63
	Klüver–Bucy Syndrome	UCV-1	PATHOPHYS-3	Neurology	17
	Knee—Anterior Cruciate Ligament Injury	UCV-1	PATHOPHYS-3	Orthopedics	72
	Knee—Combined Knee Injury	UCV-1	ANAT	Orthopedics	89
	Knee—Osgood–Schlatter's Disease	UCV-1	ANAT	Orthopedics	90
	Krabbe's Disease	UCV-1	BIOCHEM	Genetics	61
	Kwashiorkor	MC	PED	Endocrinology	306
	Kwashiorkor	UCV-1	BIOCHEM	Endocrinology	21
L	Labor and Delivery	MC	OB/GYN	Obstetrics	294
	Labyrinthitis	MC	ER	ENT/Ophthalmology	32

Case Name	SER	BOOK	SubSpecialty	Case Number
Labyrinthitis	UCV-1	PATHOPHYS-1	ENT/Ophthalmology	66
Lactase Deficiency	MC	IM-1	Gastroenterology	108
Lactic Acidosis	MC	ER	Endocrinology	23
Lactic Acidosis	UCV-1	BIOCHEM	Endocrinology	22
Laryngotracheobronchitis	MC	ER	ENT/Ophthalmology	33
Laxative Abuse	UCV-1	PHARM	Gastroenterology	30
Lead Poisoning	UCV-1	PHARM	Toxicology	101
Lead Toxicity	MC	ER	Toxicology	70
Leg—Compartment Syndrome	UCV-1	ANAT	Orthopedics	91
Legg–Calve–Perthes Disease	UCV-2	PED	Orthopedics	50
Legionella Pneumonia	UCV-1	MICRO-2	Infectious Disease	13
Legionella Pneumonia	UCV-2	IM-2	Infectious Disease	23
Leishmaniasis	UCV-1	MICRO-2	Infectious Disease	14
Leishmaniasis—Visceral	MC	IM-2	Infectious Disease	178
Leprosy	MC	IM-2	Infectious Disease	179
Leprosy—Lepromatous	UCV-1	MICRO-2	Infectious Disease	15
Leprosy—Tuberculoid	UCV-1	MICRO-2	Infectious Disease	16
Leptospirosis (Weil's Disease)	UCV-1	MICRO-2	Infectious Disease	17
Lesch–Nyhan Syndrome	UCV-1	BIOCHEM	Genetics	62
Lesch–Nyhan Syndrome	UCV-2	PED	Genetics	13
Levodopa Side Effects	UCV-1	PHARM	Neurology	67
Libman–Sacks Endocarditis	MC	IM-1	Cardiology	78
Lichen Planus	MC	IM-2	Dermatology	142
Lichen Planus	UCV-1	PATHOPHYS-1	Dermatology	39
Lidocaine Toxicity	UCV-1	PHARM	Cardiology	5
Listeria Meningitis in the Newborn	UCV-1	MICRO-2	Neonatology	79
Listeriosis	UCV-1	MICRO-2	Infectious Disease	18
Lithium Side Effects	UCV-1	PHARM	Psychopharmacology	81
Lithium Toxicity	UCV-2	PSYCH	Psychopharmacology	21
Löffler's Syndrome	MC	IM-2	Pulmonary	212
Long Thoracic Nerve Injury	UCV-1	ANAT	Neurology	64
Loop Diuretic Side Effect	UCV-1	PHARM	Nephrology/Urology	57
LSD Intoxication	UCV-2	PSYCH	Psychopharmacology	22
Lumbar Spinal Stenosis	MC	NEURO	Neurology	247
Lung Cancer—Lymphatic Metastasis	UCV-1	ANAT	Pulmonary	101
Lung Cancer—Pancoast's Syndrome	UCV-1	ANAT	Pulmonary	102
Lung Carcinoma	UCV-1	PATHOPHYS-2	Pulmonary	85
Lung Carcinoma	UCV-2	SURG	Pulmonary	50

	Case Name	SER	BOOK	SubSpecialty	Case Number
	Lung Transplant	MC	IM-2	Pulmonary	213
	Lupus Nephritis	UCV-1	PATHOPHYS-2	Nephrology/Urology	59
	Lyme Disease	UCV-1	MICRO-2	Infectious Disease	19
	Lyme Disease	UCV-2	PED	Infectious Disease	29
	Lymphatic Filariasis	UCV-1	MICRO-2	Infectious Disease	20
	Lymphocytic Choriomeningitis (LCM)	UCV-1	MICRO-2	Neurology	91
	Lymphogranuloma Venereum	MC	IM-2	Infectious Disease	180
	Lymphogranuloma Venereum	UCV-1	MICRO-2	Infectious Disease	21
M	Malaria	MC	IM-2	Infectious Disease	181
	Malaria	UCV-1	MICRO-2	Infectious Disease	22
	Male Erectile Disorder—Psychogenic	UCV-1	BEHAV-SC	Somatoform Disorders	91
	Malignant Hypertension	UCV-1	PATHOPHYS-1	Cardiology	18
	Malignant Hypertension	UCV-2	ER	Cardiology	5
	Malignant Hyperthermia	MC	NEURO	Neurology	248
	Malignant Hyperthermia	UCV-1	PHARM	Neurology	68
	Malignant Melanoma	UCV-1	PATHOPHYS-1	Dermatology	40
	Malignant Melanoma	UCV-2	SURG	Dermatology	4
	Malignant Mesothelioma	UCV-1	PATHOPHYS-2	Pulmonary	86
	Malingering	UCV-1	BEHAV-SC	Factitious Disorders	47
	Malingering	UCV-2	PSYCH	Factitious Disorder	37
	MAO—SSRI Interaction	UCV-1	PHARM	Psychopharmacology	82
	MAO Inhibitor Hypertensive Crisis	UCV-1	PHARM	Psychopharmacology	83
	MAO Inhibitor Hypertensive Crisis	UCV-2	PSYCH	Psychopharmacology	23
	Maple Syrup Urine Disease	UCV-1	BIOCHEM	Genetics	63
	Marantic Endocarditis	UCV-1	PATHOPHYS-1	Cardiology	19
	Marantic Endocarditis	UCV-2	IM-1	Cardiology	8
	Marfan's Syndrome	UCV-1	PATHOPHYS-2	Genetics	12
	Marfan's Syndrome	UCV-2	IM-2	Genetics	11
	Mass in Jugular Foramen	UCV-1	ANAT	Neurology	65
	Mastoiditis	MC	ER	ENT/Ophthalmology	34
	Maturity-Onset Diabetes of Youth	MC	IM-1	Endocrinology	92
	MDMA (Ecstasy) Toxicity	MC	ER	Psychopharm	62
	Measles	UCV-1	MICRO-2	Infectious Disease	23
	Measles	UCV-2	PED	Infectious Disease	30
	Meckel's Diverticulum	UCV-1	ANAT	General Surgery	29
	Meckel's Diverticulum	UCV-2	PED	General Surgery	10
	Meconium Aspiration	MC	PED	Neonatology	331
	Meconium Ileus	MC	PED	Neonatology	332

Case Name	SER	BOOK	SubSpecialty	Case Number
Medial Medullary Syndrome	UCV-1	ANAT	Neurology	65
Medulloblastoma	UCV-1	PATHOPHYS-3	Neurology	18
Medulloblastoma	UCV-2	NEURO	Neurology	24
Meigs' Syndrome	MC	OB/GYN	Gynecology	281
Membranoproliferative Glomerulonephritis (MPGN)	MC	IM-2	Nephrology/Urology	202
Membranoproliferative Glomerulonephritis (MPGN)	UCV-1	PATHOPHYS-2	Nephrology/Urology	60
Membranous Glomerulonephritis	UCV-1	PATHOPHYS-2	Nephrology/Urology	61
Membranous Glomerulonephritis	UCV-2	IM-2	Nephrology/Urology	35
Ménière's Disease	UCV-1	PATHOPHYS-3	Neurology	19
Ménière's Disease	UCV-2	NEURO	Neurology	25
Meningioma	MC	NEURO	Neurology	249
Meningioma	UCV-1	PATHOPHYS-3	Neurology	20
Meningitis—Aseptic	UCV-2	NEURO	Neurology	26
Meningitis—Bacterial	UCV-2	NEURO	Neurology	27
Meningitis—Bacterial (Adult)	UCV-1	MICRO-2	Neurology	92
Meningitis—Bacterial (Pediatric)	UCV-1	MICRO-2	Neurology	93
Meningitis—Cryptococcal	UCV-1	MICRO-2	Neurology	94
Meningitis—Cryptococcal	UCV-2	IM-2	Neurology	40
Meningitis—Listeria	MC	NEURO	Neurology	250
Meningitis—Tubercular	MC	NEURO	Neurology	251
Meningitis—Tubercular	UCV-1	MICRO-2	Neurology	95
Meningococcemia	UCV-1	MICRO-2	Infectious Disease	24
Meningococcemia	UCV-2	IM-2	Infectious Disease	24
Menopause	UCV-1	PATHOPHYS-3	Gynecology	52
Menopause	UCV-2	OB/GYN	Gynecology	14
Mercury Poisoning	UCV-1	PHARM	Toxicology	102
Mesenteric Adenitis	MC	SURG	General Surgery	356
Mesenteric Ischemia	UCV-1	ANAT	General Surgery	30
Mesenteric Ischemia	UCV-2	SURG	General Surgery	32
Metabolic Acidosis	MC	ER	Endocrinology	24
Metabolic Alkalosis	MC	ER	Endocrinology	25
Metabolic Alkalosis	UCV-1	BIOCHEM	Endocrinology	23
Metachromatic Leukodystrophy	UCV-1	BIOCHEM	Genetics	64
Metastatic Brain Tumor	MC	NEURO	Neurology	252
Metastatic Brain Tumor	UCV-1	PATHOPHYS-3	Neurology	21
Metastatic Carcinoma—Liver	UCV-1	PATHOPHYS-1	Gastroenterology	96

Case Name	SER	BOOK	SubSpecialty	Case Number
Methanol Poisoning	UCV-1	PHARM	Toxicology	103
Methanol Poisoning	UCV-2	ER	Toxicology	48
Methemoglobinemia	MC	IM-1	Hematology/Oncology	125
Methemoglobinemia	UCV-1	BIOCHEM	Hematology/Oncology	81
Methotrexate Toxicity	UCV-1	PHARM	Hematology/Oncology	40
Methyldopa Side Effects	UCV-1	PHARM	Cardiology	6
Methylxanthine Toxicity	MC	ER	Toxicology	71
Migraine	UCV-1	PATHOPHYS-3	Neurology	22
Migraine	UCV-2	NEURO	Neurology	28
Minimal Change Disease	UCV-1	PATHOPHYS-2	Nephrology/Urology	62
Minimal Change Disease	UCV-2	IM-2	Nephrology/Urology	36
Mitral Insufficiency	UCV-1	PATHOPHYS-1	Cardiology	20
Mitral Insufficiency	UCV-2	IM-1	Cardiology	9
Mitral Stenosis	UCV-1	PATHOPHYS-1	Cardiology	21
Mitral Stenosis	UCV-2	IM-1	Cardiology	10
Mittelschmerz	MC	OB/GYN	Gynecology	282
Mixed Connective Tissue Disorder	MC	IM-2	Rheumatology	222
Mixed Connective Tissue Disorder	UCV-1	PATHOPHYS-3	Rheumatology	83
Molluscum Contagiosum	MC	IM-2	Dermatology	143
Molluscum Contagiosum	UCV-1	MICRO-1	Dermatology	11
Monoclonal Gammopathy of Undetermined Significance	MC	IM-1	Hematology/Oncology	126
Mononeuritis Multiplex	MC	NEURO	Neurology	253
Mucormycosis	UCV-1	MICRO-2	Infectious Disease	25
Multifocal Atrial Tachycardia	MC	IM-1	Cardiology	79
Multiple Endocrine Neoplasia (MEN)	MC	IM-1	Endocrinology	93
Multiple Myeloma	UCV-1	PATHOPHYS-2	Hematology/Oncology	31
Multiple Myeloma	UCV-2	IM-1	Hematology/Oncology	50
Multiple Sclerosis	UCV-1	PATHOPHYS-3	Neurology	23
Multiple Sclerosis	UCV-2	NEURO	Neurology	29
Multisystem Organ Failure (MSOF)	MC	ER	Cardiology	10
Mumps	MC	PED	Infectious Disease	325
Mumps	UCV-1	MICRO-2	Infectious Disease	26
Munchausen's Syndrome	UCV-1	BEHAV-SC	Factitious Disorders	48
Mushroom Poisoning	UCV-1	PHARM	Toxicology	104
Myasthenia Gravis	UCV-1	PATHOPHYS-3	Neurology	24
Myasthenia Gravis	UCV-2	NEURO	Neurology	30
Mycoplasma Pneumonia	MC	IM-2	Infectious Disease	182

	Case Name	SER	BOOK	SubSpecialty	Case Number
	Mycoplasma Pneumonia	UCV-1	MICRO-2	Infectious Disease	27
	Mycosis Fungoides	UCV-1	PATHOPHYS-1	Dermatology	41
	Mycosis Fungoides—Sézary Syndrome	MC	IM-2	Dermatology	144
	Myelodysplastic Syndromes	MC	IM-1	Hematology/Oncology	27
	Myelofibrosis with Myeloid Metaplasia	UCV-1	PATHOPHYS-2	Hematology/Oncology	32
	Myocarditis	UCV-1	PATHOPHYS-1	Cardiology	22
	Myocarditis—Viral	MC	IM-1	Cardiology	80
	Myocarditis—Viral	UCV-1	MICRO-1	Cardiology	2
	Myotonic Dystrophy	UCV-1	PATHOPHYS-3	Neurology	25
	Myotonic Dystrophy	UCV-2	NEURO	Neurology	31
N	Narcissistic Personality Disorder	UCV-1	BEHAV-SC	Personality Disorders	71
	Narcolepsy	MC	NEURO	Neurology	254
	Narcolepsy	UCV-1	BEHAV-SC	Neurology	7
	Necrotizing Enterocolitis	UCV-1	MICRO-1	Gastroenterology	33
	Necrotizing Enterocolitis	UCV-2	PED	Neonatology	43
	Necrotizing Fasciitis	UCV-1	MICRO-2	Infectious Disease	28
	Neonatal Meningitis	UCV-2	PED	Neonatology	44
	Neonatal Sepsis	UCV-2	ER	Neonatology	29
	Nephrolithiasis	UCV-1	ANAT	Nephrology/Urology	47
	Nephrolithiasis	UCV-2	ER	Nephrology/Urology	30
	Nephrotic Syndrome	MC	IM-2	Nephrology/Urology	203
	Neuroblastoma	UCV-1	PATHOPHYS-3	Neurology	26
	Neuroblastoma	UCV-2	NEURO	Neurology	32
	Neurofibromatosis Type 1	MC	NEURO	Neurology	255
	Neuroleptic Malignant Syndrome	UCV-1	PHARM	Psychopharmacology	84
	Neuroleptic Malignant Syndrome	UCV-2	ER	Psychopharmacology	41
	Neurosyphilis (Tabes Dorsalis)	UCV-2	IM-2	Infectious Disease	28
	Neutropenic Enterocolitis	UCV-1	MICRO-1	Gastroenterology	34
	Nevirapine Therapy	UCV-1	PHARM	Toxicology	105
	Niacin Side Effects	UCV-1	PHARM	Cardiology	7
	Nicotine Withdrawal	UCV-1	PHARM	Psychopharmacology	85
	Niemann–Pick Disease	UCV-1	BIOCHEM	Genetics	65
	Nitrate Exposure	UCV-1	PHARM	Cardiology	8
	Nitroglycerin Tolerance	UCV-1	PHARM	Cardiology	9
	Nocardiosis	UCV-1	MICRO-2	Infectious Disease	29
	Non-Hodgkin's Lymphoma	UCV-1	PATHOPHYS-2	Hematology/Oncology	33
	Non-Hodgkin's Lymphoma	UCV-2	IM-1	Hematology/Oncology	51
	Nonketotic Hyperosmolar Coma	UCV-1	BIOCHEM	Endocrinology	24

	Case Name	SER	BOOK	SubSpecialty	Case Number
	Nonketotic Hyperosmolar Coma	UCV-2	IM-1	Endocrinology	26
	Normal Pressure Hydrocephalus	UCV-1	PATHOPHYS-3	Neurology	27
	Normal Pressure Hydrocephalus	UCV-2	NEURO	Neurology	33
	Nosocomial Enterococcal Infection	UCV-1	MICRO-2	Infectious Disease	30
	NSAID Toxicity	UCV-1	PHARM	Toxicology	106
	NSAID-Induced Qualitative Platelet Disorder	UCV-1	PHARM	Toxicology	107
	Nursemaid's Elbow	MC	ER	Orthopedics	61
O	Obsessive-Compulsive Disorder	UCV-1	BEHAV-SC	Anxiety Disorders	28
	Obsessive-Compulsive Disorder	UCV-2	PSYCH	Anxiety Disorders	7
	Obsessive-Compulsive Personality Disorder	UCV-1	BEHAV-SC	Personality Disorders	72
	Obstructive Hydrocephalus	MC	NEURO	Neurology	256
	Obstructive Hydrocephalus	UCV-1	ANAT	Neurology	67
	Obstructive Sleep Apnea	UCV-1	ANAT	Neurology	68
	Obstructive Sleep Apnea	UCV-1	PATHOPHYS-1	ENT/Ophthalmology	67
	Obstructive Sleep Apnea	UCV-2	SURG	ENT/Ophthalmology	9
	OCP-Related Cerebrovascular Accident	UCV-2	OB/GYN	Gynecology	15
	Oligodendroglioma	MC	NEURO	Neurology	257
	Oligodendroglioma	UCV-1	PATHOPHYS-3	Neurology	28
	Olivopontocerebellar Atrophy	MC	NEURO	Neurology	258
	Onchocerciasis	UCV-1	MICRO-2	Infectious Disease	31
	OPC Poisoning	UCV-1	PHARM	Toxicology	108
	OPC Poisoning	UCV-2	PED	Toxicology	56
	Open-Angle Glaucoma	UCV-1	PATHOPHYS-1	ENT/Ophthalmology	68
	Open-Angle Glaucoma	MC	IM-1	ENT/Ophthalmology	95
	Opiate Withdrawal	UCV-1	PHARM	Psychopharmacology	86
	Opiate Withdrawal	UCV-2	PSYCH	Psychopharmacology	24
	Optic Neuritis	MC	ER	ENT/Ophthalmology	35
	Oral Contraceptive Side Effects	UCV-1	PHARM	Endocrinology	18
	Orchitis	MC	SURG	Nephrology/Urology	366
	Orchitis	UCV-1	MICRO-2	Nephrology/Urology	82
	Orotic Aciduria	UCV-1	BIOCHEM	Genetics	66
	Osler–Weber–Rendu Disease (Hereditary Telangiectasia)	MC	IM-2	Dermatology	145
	Osler–Weber–Rendu Syndrome	UCV-1	PATHOPHYS-1	Dermatology	42
	Osteoarthritis	UCV-1	PATHOPHYS-3	Orthopedics	73
	Osteoarthritis	UCV-2	SURG	Orthopedics	44
	Osteogenesis Imperfecta	UCV-1	BIOCHEM	Orthopedics	89

	Case Name	SER	BOOK	SubSpecialty	Case Number
	Osteogenesis Imperfecta	UCV-2	PED	Orthopedics	52
	Osteogenic Sarcoma	UCV-1	PATHOPHYS-3	Orthopedics	74
	Osteogenic Sarcoma	UCV-2	SURG	Orthopedics	45
	Osteomalacia	UCV-1	BIOCHEM	Endocrinology	25
	Osteomalacia	UCV-2	IM-1	Endocrinology	27
	Osteomyelitis	UCV-1	MICRO-2	Orthopedics	109
	Osteomyelitis	UCV-2	SURG	Orthopedics	46
	Osteopetrosis	UCV-1	PATHOPHYS-3	Rheumatology	84
	Osteoporosis	MC	IM-2	Rheumatology	223
	Osteoporosis	UCV-1	PATHOPHYS-3	Rheumatology	85
	Osteoporosis Prophylaxis—Hormonal	UCV-1	PHARM	Endocrinology	19
	Osteoporosis Prophylaxis—Non-hormonal	UCV-1	PHARM	Endocrinology	20
	Osteoporotic Fracture—Bisphosphonates	UCV-1	PHARM	Endocrinology	21
	Otitis Externa	UCV-1	MICRO-1	ENT/Ophthalmology	23
	Otitis Externa	UCV-2	ER	ENT/Ophthalmology	11
	Otitis Media	UCV-1	MICRO-1	ENT/Ophthalmology	24
	Otitis Media—Acute	UCV-2	ER	ENT/Ophthalmology	12
	Ovarian Cancer	UCV-1	PATHOPHYS-3	Gynecology	53
	Ovarian Cancer	UCV-2	OB/GYN	Gynecology	16
	Ovarian Cyst—Corpus Luteum (Ruptured)	MC	OB/GYN	Gynecology	283
	Ovarian Cyst—Follicular	UCV-1	PATHOPHYS-3	Gynecology	54
	Ovarian Teratoma	UCV-1	PATHOPHYS-3	Gynecology	55
	Ovarian Teratoma	UCV-2	OB/GYN	Gynecology	17
	Ovarian Torsion	UCV-2	ER	Gynecology	37
	Overwhelming Postsplenectomy Infections	UCV-1	MICRO-2	Infectious Disease	32
P	Paget's Disease of Bone	MC	SURG	Orthopedics	373
	Paget's Disease of Bone	UCV-1	PATHOPHYS-3	Orthopedics	75
	Pancreatic Carcinoma	UCV-1	PATHOPHYS-2	General Surgery	10
	Pancreatic Carcinoma	UCV-2	SURG	General Surgery	33
	Pancreatic Pseudocyst	UCV-1	ANAT	Gastroenterology	20
	Pancreatic Pseudocyst	UCV-2	SURG	Gastroenterology	12
	Pancreatitis—Acute	UCV-1	PATHOPHYS-1	Gastroenterology	97
	Pancreatitis—Acute	UCV-2	SURG	Gastroenterology	13
	Panic Disorder	UCV-1	BEHAV-SC	Anxiety Disorders	29
	Panic Disorder Without Agoraphobia	UCV-2	PSYCH	Anxiety Disorders	8
	Paranoid Personality Disorder	UCV-1	BEHAV-SC	Personality Disorders	73
	Parkinson's Disease	UCV-1	ANAT	Neurology	69

Case Name	SER	BOOK	SubSpecialty	Case Number
Parkinson's Disease	UCV-2	NEURO	Neurology	34
Parkinson's Disease—MPTP-Induced	UCV-1	PHARM	Neurology	69
Parotid Gland—Pleomorphic Adenoma	MC	SURG	General Surgery	357
Paroxysmal Nocturnal Hemoglobinuria	MC	IM-1	Hematology/Oncology	128
Paroxysmal Nocturnal Hemoglobinuria	UCV-1	BIOCHEM	Hematology/Oncology	82
Paroxysmal Supraventricular Tachycardia	UCV-2	IM-1	Cardiology	11
Passive-Aggressive Personality Disorder	UCV-1	BEHAV-SC	Personality Disorders	74
Pasteurella multocida	UCV-1	MICRO-2	Infectious Disease	33
Patent Ductus Arteriosus	UCV-1	ANAT	Cardiology	6
Patent Ductus Arteriosus	UCV-2	PED	Cardiology	1
Patient Autonomy	UCV-2	PSYCH	Ethics	32
Patient-Doctor Confidentiality	UCV-2	PSYCH	Ethics	33
PCP Intoxication	UCV-1	BEHAV-SC	Psychopharmacology	97
PCP Intoxication	UCV-2	PSYCH	Psychopharmacology	25
Pediculosis	MC	IM-2	Dermatology	146
Pedophilia	UCV-1	BEHAV-SC	Paraphilia	63
Pelvic Fracture	MC	SURG	Orthopedics	374
Pelvic Fracture	UCV-1	ANAT	Orthopedics	92
Pelvic Inflammatory Disease	UCV-1	MICRO-2	Gynecology	104
Pelvic Inflammatory Disease	UCV-2	OB/GYN	Gynecology	18
Pelvic Tuberculosis	UCV-1	MICRO-2	Gynecology	105
Pelvic Tuberculosis	UCV-2	OB/GYN	Gynecology	19
Pemphigus	MC	ER	Dermatology	19
Pemphigus	UCV-1	PATHOPHYS-1	Dermatology	43
Penetrating Anterior Abdominal Wound	UCV-2	ER	General Surgery	18
Penetrating Thoracic Injury	UCV-2	ER	General Surgery	19
Penicillin Allergic Reaction	UCV-1	PHARM	Infectious Disease	52
Peptic Ulcer—Perforated	UCV-2	SURG	Gastroenterology	14
Peptic Ulcer—Perforated	UCV-1	ANAT	Gastroenterology	21
Peptic Ulcer Disease	UCV-2	IM-1	Gastroenterology	38
Peptic Ulcer Disease *(H pylori)*	UCV-1	MICRO-1	Gastroenterology	35
Perianal Abscess	MC	SURG	General Surgery	358
Pericardial Effusion	MC	IM-1	Cardiology	81
Pericarditis	UCV-2	IM-1	Cardiology	12
Pericarditis—Acute	UCV-1	MICRO-1	Cardiology	3
Peripheral Arterial Embolism	UCV-1	PATHOPHYS-1	Cardiology	23
Peripheral Neuropathy—Diabetic	MC	NEURO	Neurology	259
Peripheral Neuropathy—Diabetic	UCV-1	PATHOPHYS-3	Neurology	29

Case Name	SER	BOOK	SubSpecialty	Case Number
Peripheral Neuropathy due to Vincristine	UCV-2	NEURO	Neurology	35
Peritonsillar Abscess	MC	ER	ENT/Ophthalmology	36
Petit's Triangle Hernia	MC	SURG	General Surgery	359
Petit's Triangle Hernia	UCV-1	ANAT	General Surgery	31
Peutz–Jeghers Syndrome	UCV-1	PATHOPHYS-1	Gastroenterology	98
Pharyngitis—Adenoviral	MC	IM-1	ENT/Ophthalmology	96
Pharyngitis—Adenovirus	UCV-1	MICRO-1	ENT/Ophthalmology	25
Pharyngitis—Streptococcal	MC	IM-1	ENT/Ophthalmology	97
Pharyngitis—Streptococcal	UCV-1	MICRO-1	ENT/Ophthalmology	26
Phenylketonuria (PKU)	UCV-1	BIOCHEM	Genetics	67
Phenylketonuria (PKU)	UCV-2	PED	Genetics	14
Phenytoin Overdose	UCV-1	PHARM	Neurology	70
Pheochromocytoma	UCV-1	BIOCHEM	Endocrinology	26
Pheochromocytoma	UCV-2	SURG	Endocrinology	7
Phosphoenolpyruvate Carboxykinase Deficiency	UCV-1	BIOCHEM	Genetics	68
Physiologic Jaundice Of Newborn	UCV-2	PED	Neonatology	45
Pick's Disease	UCV-2	NEURO	Neurology	36
Pilonidal Cyst	MC	SURG	General Surgery	360
Pinealoma	UCV-1	PATHOPHYS-1	Endocrinology	58
Pinworm Infection	UCV-1	MICRO-1	Gastroenterology	36
Pityriasis Alba	MC	PED	Dermatology	301
Pityriasis Rosea	MC	IM-2	Dermatology	147
Pityriasis Rosea	UCV-1	PATHOPHYS-1	Dermatology	44
Pityriasis Versicolor	MC	IM-2	Dermatology	148
Pityriasis Versicolor	UCV-1	MICRO-1	Dermatology	12
Placenta Previa	UCV-2	OB/GYN	Obstetrics	43
Placental Abruption	UCV-2	OB/GYN	Obstetrics	44
Plague	UCV-1	MICRO-2	Infectious Disease	34
Pleural Effusion	UCV-1	PATHOPHYS-2	Pulmonary	87
Plummer–Vinson Syndrome	UCV-1	PATHOPHYS-1	Gastroenterology	99
Plummer–Vinson Syndrome	UCV-2	SURG	Gastroenterology	15
Pneumococcal Pneumonia	UCV-1	MICRO-2	Infectious Disease	35
Pneumococcal Pneumonia	UCV-2	IM-2	Infectious Disease	25
Pneumocystis carinii Pneumonia	UCV-1	MICRO-2	Infectious Disease	36
Pneumothorax—Open	MC	ER	Pulmonary	65
Pneumothorax—Spontaneous	UCV-2	IM-2	Pulmonary	47
Pneumothorax—Spontaneous	UCV-1	PATHOPHYS-2	Pulmonary	88
Pneumothorax—Tension	UCV-2	SURG	Pulmonary	51

Case Name	SER	BOOK	SubSpecialty	Case Number
Pneumothorax—Tension	UCV-1	PATHOPHYS-2	Pulmonary	89
Poliomyelitis	UCV-1	MICRO-2	Neurology	96
Poliomyelitis	UCV-2	NEURO	Neurology	37
Polyarteritis Nodosa	UCV-1	PATHOPHYS-3	Rheumatology	86
Polyarteritis Nodosa	UCV-2	IM-2	Rheumatology	53
Polycystic Ovary Disease	UCV-1	PATHOPHYS-3	Gynecology	56
Polycystic Ovary Disease	UCV-2	OB/GYN	Gynecology	20
Polycythemia Vera (PCV)	UCV-1	PATHOPHYS-2	Hematology/Oncology	34
Polycythemia Vera (PCV)	UCV-2	IM-1	Hematology/Oncology	52
Polyhydramnios	UCV-2	OB/GYN	Obstetrics	45
Polymyalgia Rheumatica	MC	IM-2	Rheumatology	224
Polymyalgia Rheumatica	UCV-1	PATHOPHYS-3	Rheumatology	87
Polymyositis	MC	IM-2	Rheumatology	225
Polymyositis	UCV-1	PATHOPHYS-3	Rheumatology	88
Pompe's Disease	UCV-1	BIOCHEM	Genetics	69
Popliteal Fossa Trauma	UCV-1	ANAT	General Surgery	32
Porphyria Cutanea Tarda	MC	IM-2	Genetics	156
Porphyria Cutanea Tarda	UCV-1	BIOCHEM	Genetics	70
Portal Hypertension	UCV-1	ANAT	Gastroenterology	22
Portal Hypertension	UCV-2	SURG	Gastroenterology	16
Portal Vein Thrombosis	UCV-2	PED	Gastroenterology	8
Port-Wine Stain	MC	SURG	Dermatology	337
Postpartum Hemorrhage	MC	OB/GYN	Obstetrics	295
Postpartum Hemorrhage	UCV-1	PATHOPHYS-3	Obstetrics	64
Postpartum Thrombophlebitis	UCV-1	PATHOPHYS-3	Obstetrics	65
Poststreptococcal Glomerulonephritis	UCV-1	MICRO-2	Nephrology/Urology	83
Poststreptococcal Glomerulonephritis	UCV-2	PED	Nephrology/Urology	47
Post-Traumatic Stress Disorder	UCV-1	BEHAV-SC	Anxiety Disorders	30
Post-Traumatic Stress Disorder	UCV-2	PSYCH	Anxiety Disorders	9
Post-Traumatic Stress Disorder (Child)	UCV-1	BEHAV-SC	Child Psychiatry	37
Precocious Puberty	MC	PED	Endocrinology	307
Precocious Puberty	UCV-1	BIOCHEM	Endocrinology	27
Pregnancy with IUD	UCV-2	OB/GYN	Obstetrics	46
Premenstrual Dysphoric Disorder	UCV-1	BEHAV-SC	Mood Disorders	59
Premenstrual Dysphoric Disorder	UCV-2	OB/GYN	Gynecology	21
Presbycusis	UCV-1	PATHOPHYS-1	ENT/Ophthalmology	69
Presbyopia	UCV-1	PATHOPHYS-1	ENT/Ophthalmology	70
Primary Amenorrhea—Testicular Feminization	UCV-1	BIOCHEM	Gynecology	87

Case Name	SER	BOOK	SubSpecialty	Case Number
Primary Amenorrhea—Testicular Feminization	UCV-2	OB/GYN	Gynecology	22
Primary Amenorrhea—Turner's Syndrome	UCV-1	PATHOPHYS-3	Gynecology	57
Primary Amenorrhea—Turner's Syndrome	UCV-2	OB/GYN	Gynecology	23
Primary Biliary Cirrhosis	UCV-1	PATHOPHYS-1	Gastroenterology	100
Primary Biliary Cirrhosis	UCV-2	IM-1	Gastroenterology	39
Primary Insomnia	UCV-1	BEHAV-SC	Sleep Disorders	86
Primary Pulmonary Hypertension	MC	IM-2	Pulmonary	214
Primary Pulmonary Hypertension	UCV-1	PATHOPHYS-2	Pulmonary	90
Primary Sclerosing Cholangitis	MC	IM-1	Gastroenterology	109
Proctocolitis	MC	IM-2	Infectious Disease	183
Proctocolitis	UCV-1	MICRO-2	Infectious Disease	37
Progressive Multifocal Leukoencephalopathy	MC	NEURO	Neurology	260
Progressive Multifocal Leukoencephalopathy	UCV-1	MICRO-2	Neurology	97
Progressive Systemic Sclerosis (Scleroderma)	MC	IM-2	Rheumatology	226
Progressive Systemic Sclerosis (Scleroderma)	UCV-1	PATHOPHYS-3	Rheumatology	89
Prolactinoma	UCV-1	PATHOPHYS-1	Endocrinology	59
Prostate Carcinoma	UCV-1	PATHOPHYS-2	Nephrology/Urology	63
Prostate Carcinoma	UCV-2	SURG	Nephrology/Urology	37
Prostatitis—Acute	UCV-1	MICRO-2	Nephrology/Urology	84
Prostatitis—Chronic	UCV-1	MICRO-2	Nephrology/Urology	85
Prosthetic Valve Endocarditis	MC	ER	Cardiology	11
Prosthetic Valve Endocarditis	UCV-1	MICRO-1	Cardiology	4
Protease Inhibitor Side Effects	UCV-1	PHARM	Toxicology	109
Pseudobulbar Palsy	MC	NEURO	Neurology	261
Pseudobulbar Palsy	UCV-1	PATHOPHYS-3	Neurology	30
Pseudocyesis	UCV-1	BEHAV-SC	Somatoform Disorders	92
Pseudodementia	MC	NEURO	Psychiatry-Mood Disorders	269
Pseudogout	MC	SURG	Rheumatology	380
Pseudogout	UCV-1	PATHOPHYS-3	Rheumatology	90
Pseudohyperkalemia	MC	ER	Endocrinology	26
Pseudohypoparathyroidism	UCV-1	BIOCHEM	Endocrinology	28
Pseudomembranous Colitis	MC	IM-1	Gastroenterology	110
Pseudomembranous Colitis	UCV-1	PHARM	Gastroenterology	31
Pseudoseizures	MC	NEURO	Psychiatry-Factitious Disorders	268
Pseudotumor Cerebri	UCV-1	PATHOPHYS-1	ENT/Ophthalmology	71
Pseudotumor Cerebri	UCV-2	NEURO	Neurology	38
Psittacosis	UCV-1	MICRO-2	Infectious Disease	38
Psoriasis	UCV-1	PATHOPHYS-1	Dermatology	45

	Case Name	SER	BOOK	SubSpecialty	Case Number
	Psoriasis	UCV-2	IM-2	Dermatology	8
	Psoriatic Arthritis	MC	IM-2	Rheumatology	227
	Pudendal Nerve Block	UCV-1	ANAT	Obstetrics	75
	Puerperal Sepsis	UCV-2	OB/GYN	Obstetrics	47
	Pulmonary Embolism	UCV-1	PATHOPHYS-2	Pulmonary	91
	Pulmonary Embolism	UCV-2	ER	Pulmonary	46
	Pulmonary Eosinophilia Syndromes	MC	IM-2	Pulmonary	215
	Pulmonic Stenosis	UCV-2	PED	Cardiology	2
	Pyelonephritis—Acute	UCV-1	MICRO-2	Nephrology/Urology	86
	Pyelonephritis—Acute	UCV-2	ER	Nephrology/Urology	31
	Pyoderma Gangrenosum	MC	IM-2	Dermatology	149
	Pyoderma Gangrenosum	UCV-1	PATHOPHYS-1	Dermatology	46
	Pyogenic Granuloma	MC	IM-2	Infectious Disease	184
	Pyogenic Liver Abscess	MC	ER	Infectious Disease	58
	Pyogenic Liver Abscess	UCV-1	MICRO-2	Infectious Disease	39
	Pyruvate Kinase Deficiency	UCV-1	BIOCHEM	Genetics	71
Q	Q Fever	MC	IM-2	Infectious Disease	185
	Q Fever	UCV-1	MICRO-2	Infectious Disease	40
	Quinidine Side Effects	UCV-1	PHARM	Cardiology	10
R	Rabies	MC	NEURO	Infectious Disease	231
	Rabies	UCV-1	MICRO-2	Infectious Disease	41
	Ramsay Hunt Syndrome	UCV-1	MICRO-2	Neurology	98
	Ramsay Hunt Syndrome	UCV-2	NEURO	Neurology	39
	Rape	UCV-2	OB/GYN	Gynecology	24
	Rat Bite Fever	UCV-1	MICRO-2	Infectious Disease	42
	Rationalization	UCV-1	BEHAV-SC	Defense Mechanism	20
	Raynaud's Disease	UCV-1	PATHOPHYS-3	Rheumatology	91
	Reaction Formation	UCV-1	BEHAV-SC	Defense Mechanism	21
	Recurrent Laryngeal Nerve Lesion	UCV-1	ANAT	Neurology	70
	Reflex Sympathetic Dystrophy	MC	SURG	Orthopedics	375
	Regression	UCV-1	BEHAV-SC	Defense Mechanism	22
	Reiter's Syndrome	UCV-1	PATHOPHYS-3	Rheumatology	92
	Reiter's Syndrome	UCV-2	IM-2	Rheumatology	54
	Relapsing Fever	UCV-1	MICRO-2	Infectious Disease	43
	Renal Cell Carcinoma	UCV-1	PATHOPHYS-2	Nephrology/Urology	64
	Renal Cell Carcinoma	UCV-2	SURG	Nephrology/Urology	38
	Renal Infarction	UCV-1	PATHOPHYS-2	Nephrology/Urology	65
	Renal Papillary Necrosis	UCV-1	PHARM	Nephrology/Urology	58

Case Name	SER	BOOK	SubSpecialty	Case Number
Renal Transplant	MC	IM-2	Nephrology/Urology	204
Renal Tubular Acidosis	UCV-1	BIOCHEM	Nephrology/Urology	83
Renal Tubular Acidosis	UCV-2	IM-2	Nephrology/Urology	37
Renovascular Hypertension	UCV-1	PATHOPHYS-2	Nephrology/Urology	66
Renovascular Hypertension—Fibromuscular Dysplasia	UCV-2	IM-2	Nephrology/Urology	38
Repression	UCV-1	BEHAV-SC	Defense Mechanism	23
Respiratory Acidosis	MC	ER	Endocrinology	27
Respiratory Alkalosis	MC	ER	Endocrinology	28
Restraints	MC	NEURO	Psychiatry– Ethics	267
Restrictive Cardiomyopathy	MC	IM-1	Cardiology	82
Retinal Detachment	MC	ER	ENT/Ophthalmology	42
Retinitis Pigmentosa	UCV-1	PATHOPHYS-1	ENT/Ophthalmology	72
Retinoblastoma	MC	PED	ENT/Ophthalmology	310
Retinoblastoma	UCV-1	PATHOPHYS-1	ENT/Ophthalmology	73
Reversal of Tubal Ligation	UCV-2	OB/GYN	Gynecology	25
Reye's Syndrome	UCV-1	PHARM	Gastroenterology	32
Reye's Syndrome	UCV-2	ER	Gastroenterology	14
Rh Incompatibility	MC	OB/GYN	Hematology/Oncology	271
Rhabdomyolysis	MC	ER	Nephrology/Urology	60
Rhabdomyolysis	UCV-1	BIOCHEM	Nephrology/Urology	84
Rheumatic Heart Disease	UCV-2	IM-1	Cardiology	13
Rheumatoid Arthritis	UCV-1	PATHOPHYS-3	Rheumatology	93
Rheumatoid Arthritis	UCV-2	IM-2	Rheumatology	55
Richter's Hernia	MC	SURG	General Surgery	361
Richter's Hernia	UCV-1	ANAT	General Surgery	33
Rickets	MC	PED	Endocrinology	308
Rickets	UCV-1	BIOCHEM	Endocrinology	29
Rifampin Side Effects	UCV-1	PHARM	Infectious Disease	53
Rocky Mountain Spotted Fever	UCV-1	MICRO-2	Infectious Disease	44
Rocky Mountain Spotted Fever	UCV-2	PED	Infectious Disease	31
Roseola Infantum	UCV-1	MICRO-1	Dermatology	13
Roseola Infantum (Exanthem Subitum)	MC	PED	Dermatology	302
Rotavirus Diarrhea in Infants	UCV-1	MICRO-1	Gastroenterology	37
RSV Pneumonia	UCV-1	MICRO-2	Infectious Disease	45
Rubella—Congenital	MC	PED	Infectious Disease	326
Rubella—Congenital	UCV-1	MICRO-2	Infectious Disease	46
Rubella—Congenital	UCV-2	OB/GYN	Obstetrics	48

	Case Name	SER	BOOK	SubSpecialty	Case Number
	Rubella (German Measles)	UCV-1	MICRO-2	Infectious Disease	47
	Rubella (German Measles)	UCV-2	IM-2	Infectious Disease	26
S	Salicylate Toxicity	UCV-1	PHARM	Toxicology	110
	Salicylate Toxicity	UCV-2	ER	Toxicology	49
	Salmonella Food Poisoning	UCV-1	MICRO-1	Gastroenterology	38
	Salmonella Septicemia with Osteomyelitis	UCV-1	MICRO-2	Infectious Disease	48
	Sarcoidosis	UCV-1	PATHOPHYS-2	Pulmonary	92
	Sarcoidosis	UCV-2	IM-2	Pulmonary	48
	Sarcoma Botryoides	UCV-1	PATHOPHYS-2	Hematology/Oncology	35
	Scabies	MC	IM-2	Infectious Disease	186
	Scabies	UCV-1	MICRO-2	Infectious Disease	49
	Scalded Skin Syndrome	MC	PED	Dermatology	303
	Scalded Skin Syndrome	UCV-1	MICRO-1	Dermatology	14
	Scarlet Fever	MC	IM-2	Infectious Disease	187
	Scarlet Fever	UCV-1	MICRO-2	Infectious Disease	50
	Schistosomiasis	UCV-1	MICRO-2	Infectious Disease	51
	Schistosomiasis—Urinary	UCV-1	MICRO-2	Infectious Disease	52
	Schizoid Personality Disorder	UCV-1	BEHAV-SC	Personality Disorders	75
	Schizoid Personality Disorder	UCV-2	PSYCH	Personality Disorders	46
	Schizophrenia	UCV-2	PSYCH	Psychotic Disorders	49
	Schizophrenia—Acute	UCV-1	BEHAV-SC	Psychotic Disorders	80
	Schizophrenia—Catatonic	UCV-1	BEHAV-SC	Psychotic Disorders	81
	Schizophrenia—Disorganized	UCV-1	BEHAV-SC	Psychotic Disorders	82
	Schizophrenia—Paranoid	UCV-1	BEHAV-SC	Psychotic Disorders	83
	Schizophrenia—Residual	UCV-1	BEHAV-SC	Psychotic Disorders	84
	Schizophreniform Disorder	UCV-1	BEHAV-SC	Psychotic Disorders	85
	Schizotypal Personality Disorder	UCV-1	BEHAV-SC	Personality Disorders	76
	Scoliosis	MC	SURG	General Surgery	362
	Seborrheic Dermatitis	UCV-1	PATHOPHYS-1	Dermatology	47
	Seborrheic Dermatitis	UCV-2	IM-2	Dermatology	9
	Seborrheic Keratosis	MC	IM-2	Dermatology	150
	Secondary Amenorrhea	UCV-1	BIOCHEM	Gynecology	88
	Secondary Amenorrhea—Prolactinoma	UCV-2	OB/GYN	Gynecology	26
	Seizure, Absence	UCV-1	BEHAV-SC	Neurology	8
	Seizure, Absence	UCV-2	NEURO	Neurology	40
	Seizure, Complex Partial	UCV-2	NEURO	Neurology	41
	Seizure, Febrile	UCV-2	NEURO	Neurology	42
	Seizure, Grand Mal	UCV-1	BEHAV-SC	Neurology	9

Case Name	SER	BOOK	SubSpecialty	Case Number
Seizure, Grand Mal	UCV-2	NEURO	Neurology	43
Seizure, Jacksonian Type	UCV-1	BEHAV-SC	Neurology	10
Seizure, Metastatic Disease	UCV-2	NEURO	Neurology	44
Seizure, Temporal Lobe	UCV-1	BEHAV-SC	Neurology	11
Selective IgA Deficiency	UCV-1	MICRO-2	Immunology	4
Seminoma	UCV-1	PATHOPHYS-2	Nephrology/Urology	67
Seminoma	UCV-2	SURG	Nephrology/Urology	39
Separation Anxiety	UCV-1	BEHAV-SC	Child Psychiatry	38
Septic Arthritis—Gonococcal	UCV-1	MICRO-2	Orthopedics	110
Septic Arthritis—Staphylococcal	UCV-1	PATHOPHYS-3	Orthopedics	76
Septic Arthritis—Staphylococcal	UCV-2	IM-2	Orthopedics	41
Serum Sickness	UCV-1	PATHOPHYS-2	Immunology	44
Severe Combined Immunodeficiency (SCID)	UCV-1	MICRO-2	Immunology	5
Severe Combined Immunodeficiency	UCV-2	PED	Immunology	37
Sexual Masochism	UCV-1	BEHAV-SC	Paraphilia	64
Sexual Sadism	UCV-1	BEHAV-SC	PARAPHILIA	65
Sheehan's Syndrome	UCV-1	PATHOPHYS-3	Obstetrics	66
Sheehan's Syndrome	UCV-2	OB/GYN	Obstetrics	49
Shigellosis	MC	IM-2	Infectious Disease	188
Shigellosis	UCV-1	MICRO-2	Infectious Disease	53
Shock—Hypovolemic	MC	ER	Cardiology	12
Shock—Hypovolemic	UCV-1	PATHOPHYS-1	Cardiology	24
Shock—Septic	UCV-1	MICRO-2	Infectious Disease	54
Shock—Septic	UCV-2	ER	Infectious Disease	26
Shoulder Dislocation	UCV-1	ANAT	Orthopedics	93
Shoulder Dislocation	UCV-2	SURG	Orthopedics	47
Shoulder Separation	UCV-1	ANAT	Orthopedics	94
Shy–Drager Syndrome	MC	NEURO	Neurology	262
SIADH	UCV-1	BIOCHEM	Endocrinology	30
SIADH	UCV-2	IM-1	Endocrinology	28
Sialolithiasis	UCV-1	ANAT	ENT/Ophthalmology	12
Sickle Cell Anemia	UCV-1	PATHOPHYS-2	Hematology/Oncology	36
Sickle Cell Anemia	UCV-2	PED	Hematology/Oncology	21
Sickle Cell Anemia—Vaso-occlusive Crisis	UCV-2	ER	Hematology/Oncology	23
Sideroblastic Anemia	MC	IM-1	Hematology/Oncology	129
Sigmoid Volvulus	UCV-1	ANAT	General Surgery	34
Sigmoid Volvulus	UCV-2	ER	General Surgery	20
Silicosis	UCV-1	PATHOPHYS-2	Pulmonary	93

Case Name	SER	BOOK	SubSpecialty	Case Number
Silicosis	UCV-2	IM-2	Pulmonary	49
Sinus Bradycardia	UCV-1	PATHOPHYS-1	Cardiology	25
Sjögren's Syndrome	MC	IM-2	Rheumatology	228
Sjögren's Syndrome	UCV-1	PATHOPHYS-3	Rheumatology	94
Sleep Terrors	UCV-1	BEHAV-SC	Child Psychiatry	39
Sleep Terrors	UCV-2	PSYCH	Child	15
Sleepwalking Disorder	UCV-1	BEHAV-SC	Sleep Disorders	87
Smoking During Pregnancy	UCV-2	OB/GYN	Obstetrics	50
Social Phobia	UCV-1	BEHAV-SC	Anxiety Disorders	31
Social Phobia	UCV-2	PSYCH	Anxiety Disorders	10
Somatization Disorder	UCV-1	BEHAV-SC	Somatoform Disorders	93
Somatization Disorder	UCV-2	PSYCH	Somatoform Disorders	53
Somatoform Pain Disorder	UCV-1	BEHAV-SC	Somatoform Disorders	94
Spider Bite—Brown Recluse	MC	ER	Toxicology	72
Spider Bite—Widow	MC	ER	Toxicology	73
Spina Bifida	MC	NEURO	Neurology	263
Spina Bifida	UCV-1	ANAT	Neurology	71
Spinal Cord Injury	UCV-2	NEURO	Neurology	45
Spine—Cervical Spondylosis	UCV-1	PATHOPHYS-3	Orthopedics	77
Spine—Low Back Pain	UCV-2	SURG	Orthopedics	48
Spine—Prolapsed Intervertebral Disc	MC	SURG	Orthopedics	376
Spine—Prolapsed Intervertebral Disc	UCV-1	ANAT	Orthopedics	95
Spine—Spondylolisthesis	MC	SURG	Orthopedics	377
Splenic Rupture	UCV-1	ANAT	General Surgery	35
Splenic Rupture	UCV-2	SURG	General Surgery	34
Splitting	UCV-1	BEHAV-SC	Defense Mechanism	24
Spontaneous Bacterial Peritonitis	MC	ER	Gastroenterology	52
Spontaneous Bacterial Peritonitis	UCV-1	MICRO-1	Gastroenterology	39
Sporadic Multinodular Goiter	UCV-1	PATHOPHYS-1	Endocrinology	60
Sporotrichosis	UCV-1	MICRO-2	Infectious Disease	55
Squamous Cell Carcinoma	UCV-2	IM-2	Dermatology	10
Squamous Cell Carcinoma—Lip	UCV-1	ANAT	Dermatology	41
St Louis Encephalitis	UCV-1	MICRO-2	Neurology	99
Status Epilepticus	UCV-1	BEHAV-SC	Neurology	12
Status Epilepticus	UCV-2	ER	Neurology	34
Stevens–Johnson Syndrome	UCV-1	PHARM	Dermatology	12
Stevens–Johnson Syndrome	UCV-2	ER	Dermatology	7
Straddle Injury	UCV-1	ANAT	General Surgery	36

	Case Name	SER	BOOK	SubSpecialty	Case Number
	Strangulated Femoral Hernia	UCV-2	SURG	General Surgery	23
	Strongyloidiasis	UCV-1	MICRO-2	Infectious Disease	56
	Stye	MC	ER	ENT/Ophthalmology	43
	Subacute Bacterial Endocarditis	UCV-1	MICRO-1	Cardiology	5
	Subacute Bacterial Endocarditis	UCV-2	IM-2	Cardiology	2
	Subacute Sclerosing Panencephalitis	UCV-1	MICRO-2	Neurology	100
	Subacute Sclerosing Panencephalitis	UCV-2	NEURO	Neurology	46
	Subarachnoid Hemorrhage	MC	NEURO	Neurology	264
	Subarachnoid Hemorrhage	UCV-1	PATHOPHYS-3	Neurology	31
	Subdiaphragmatic Abscess	UCV-1	MICRO-2	Infectious Disease	57
	Subdural Hematoma	UCV-1	PATHOPHYS-3	Neurology	32
	Subdural Hematoma—Acute	UCV-2	ER	Neurology	35
	Sublimation	UCV-1	BEHAV-SC	Defense Mechanism	25
	Sudden Infant Death Syndrome (SIDS)	UCV-1	PATHOPHYS-2	Neonatology	47
	Sudden Infant Death Syndrome	UCV-2	PED	Neonatology	46
	Superior Vena Cava Syndrome	MC	ER	Cardiology	13
	Suppurative Hidradenitis	UCV-2	SURG	Dermatology	5
	Syphilis—Congenital	UCV-1	MICRO-2	Infectious Disease	58
	Syphilis—Congenital	UCV-2	PED	Infectious Disease	32
	Syphilis—Primary	MC	IM-2	Infectious Disease	189
	Syphilis—Primary	UCV-1	MICRO-2	Infectious Disease	59
	Syphilis—Secondary	UCV-1	MICRO-2	Infectious Disease	60
	Syphilis—Secondary	UCV-2	IM-2	Infectious Disease	27
	Syphilis—Tertiary (Aortitis)	MC	IM-2	Infectious Disease	190
	Syphilis—Tertiary (Aortitis)	UCV-1	PATHOPHYS-2	Infectious Disease	45
	Syphilis—Tertiary (Tabes Dorsalis)	UCV-1	MICRO-2	Infectious Disease	61
	Syringomyelia	MC	NEURO	Neurology	265
	Syringomyelia	UCV-1	PATHOPHYS-3	Neurology	33
	Systemic Lupus Erythematosus (SLE)	UCV-1	PATHOPHYS-3	Rheumatology	95
	Systemic Lupus Erythematosus (SLE)	UCV-2	IM-2	Rheumatology	56
T	Takayasu's Arteritis	MC	IM-2	Rheumatology	229
	Tamiflu (Oseltamivir) Therapy	UCV-1	PHARM	Infectious Disease	54
	Tarasoff's Decision	UCV-2	PSYCH	Ethics	34
	Tardive Dyskinesia	UCV-1	PHARM	Psychopharmacology	87
	Tardive Dyskinesia	UCV-2	PSYCH	Psychopharmacology	26
	Tay–Sachs Disease	UCV-1	BIOCHEM	Genetics	72
	Temporal Arteritis (Giant Cell Arteritis)	UCV-1	PATHOPHYS-3	Neurology	34

Case Name	SER	BOOK	SubSpecialty	Case Number
Temporal Arteritis (Giant Cell Arteritis)	UCV-2	NEURO	Neurology	47
Temporomandibular Joint Dislocation	UCV-1	ANAT	Orthopedics	96
Temporomandibular Joint Syndrome	MC	IM-2	Rheumatology	230
Tension Headache	UCV-2	NEURO	Neurology	48
Testicular Choriocarcinoma	UCV-1	PATHOPHYS-2	Nephrology/Urology	68
Testicular Dysgenesis	MC	PED	Nephrology/Urology	334
Testicular Dysgenesis	UCV-1	PATHOPHYS-2	Nephrology/Urology	69
Testicular Teratoma	UCV-1	PATHOPHYS-2	Nephrology/Urology	70
Testicular Torsion	UCV-1	PATHOPHYS-2	Nephrology/Urology	71
Testicular Torsion	UCV-2	ER	Nephrology/Urology	32
Testosterone Deficiency	UCV-1	PHARM	Endocrinology	22
Tetanus	MC	NEURO	Infectious Disease	232
Tetanus	UCV-1	MICRO-2	Infectious Disease	62
Tetanus Neonatorum	UCV-1	MICRO-2	Infectious Disease	63
Tetanus Neonatorum	UCV-2	PED	Infectious Disease	33
Tetracycline Rash	UCV-1	PHARM	Infectious Disease	55
Tetralogy of Fallot	UCV-1	ANAT	Cardiology	7
Tetralogy of Fallot	UCV-2	SURG	Cardiology	3
Thalassemia—Alpha	UCV-2	IM-1	Hematology/Oncology	53
Thalassemia—Beta	MC	PED	Hematology/Oncology	322
Thalassemia—Beta	UCV-1	PATHOPHYS-2	Hematology/Oncology	37
Thalidomide Exposure	UCV-1	PHARM	Toxicology	111
Thermal Burns	UCV-2	ER	General Surgery	21
Thiazide Side Effects	UCV-1	PHARM	Nephrology/Urology	59
Thioridazine Side Effects	UCV-1	PHARM	Psychopharmacology	88
Thoracic Aortic Aneurysm	MC	ER	Cardiology	14
Thorax—Cervical Rib	UCV-1	ANAT	Orthopedics	97
Thromboangiitis Obliterans (Buerger's Disease)	UCV-1	PATHOPHYS-1	Cardiology	26
Thrombophlebitis—Superficial	MC	IM-1	Cardiology	83
Thrombophlebitis—Superficial	UCV-1	PATHOPHYS-1	Cardiology	27
Thrombotic Thrombocytopenic Purpura	UCV-1	PATHOPHYS-2	Hematology/Oncology	38
Thrombotic Thrombocytopenic Purpura	UCV-2	IM-1	Hematology/Oncology	54
Thyroglossal Duct Cyst	UCV-1	ANAT	ENT/Ophthalmology	13
Thyroid Carcinoma	UCV-1	PATHOPHYS-1	Endocrinology	61
Thyroid Carcinoma	UCV-2	SURG	Endocrinology	8
Thyroid Storm	UCV-1	BIOCHEM	Endocrinology	31
Thyroid Storm	UCV-2	ER	Endocrinology	9

Case Name	SER	BOOK	SubSpecialty	Case Number
Tic Disorder—Tourette's	UCV-1	BEHAV-SC	Child Psychiatry	40
Tic Disorder—Transient	UCV-2	PSYCH	Child	16
Tick Paralysis	UCV-1	MICRO-2	Infectious Disease	64
Tietze's Syndrome	MC	ER	Cardiology	15
Tinea Corporis (Ringworm)	MC	IM-2	Dermatology	151
Tinea Corporis (Ringworm)	UCV-1	MICRO-1	Dermatology	15
Todd's Paralysis	MC	NEURO	Neurology	266
Tonsillitis	UCV-1	ANAT	ENT/Ophthalmology	14
Torsades de Pointes	UCV-2	IM-1	Cardiology	14
Torsion of the Appendix Testis	MC	SURG	Nephrology/Urology	367
Toxemia of Pregnancy—Eclampsia	UCV-2	OB/GYN	Obstetrics	51
Toxemia of Pregnancy—Preeclampsia	UCV-1	PATHOPHYS-3	Obstetrics	67
Toxic Epidermal Necrolysis	MC	ER	Dermatology	20
Toxic Megacolon	MC	SURG	Gastroenterology	342
Toxic Megacolon	UCV-1	PATHOPHYS-1	Gastroenterology	101
Toxic Shock Syndrome (TSS)	UCV-1	MICRO-2	Gynecology	106
Toxic Shock Syndrome (TSS)	UCV-2	OB/GYN	Gynecology	27
Toxoplasmosis	MC	IM-2	Infectious Disease	191
Toxoplasmosis	UCV-1	MICRO-2	Infectious Disease	65
Toxoplasmosis—Congenital	UCV-2	PED	Infectious Disease	34
Tracheoesophageal Fistula	MC	PED	Gastroenterology	313
Tracheoesophageal Fistula	UCV-1	ANAT	Gastroenterology	23
Transfusion Reaction—Acute Hemolytic	UCV-1	PATHOPHYS-2	Hematology/Oncology	39
Transfusion Reaction—Febrile Nonhemolytic	UCV-1	PATHOPHYS-2	Hematology/Oncology	40
Transfusion Reaction—Hemolytic	MC	ER	Hematology/Oncology	56
Transient Ischemic Attack	UCV-2	ER	Neurology	36
Traveler's Diarrhea	UCV-1	MICRO-1	Gastroenterology	40
Trichinosis	MC	IM-2	Infectious Disease	192
Trichinosis	UCV-1	MICRO-2	Infectious Disease	66
Tricyclic Antidepressant Overdose	UCV-1	PHARM	Psychopharmacology	89
Tricyclic Antidepressant Overdose	UCV-2	ER	Psychopharmacology	42
Trigeminal Neuralgia	UCV-1	ANAT	Neurology	72
Trigeminal Neuralgia	UCV-2	NEURO	Neurology	49
Tuberculosis—Miliary	UCV-1	MICRO-2	Infectious Disease	67
Tuberculosis—Pulmonary	UCV-1	MICRO-2	Infectious Disease	68
Tuberculosis—Pulmonary	UCV-2	IM-2	Infectious Disease	29
Tubo-Ovarian Abscess	MC	OB/GYN	Gynecology	284
Tubulointerstitial Disease—Drug-Induced	UCV-1	PHARM	Nephrology/Urology	60

	Case Name	SER	BOOK	SubSpecialty	Case Number
	Tularemia	MC	IM-2	Infectious Disease	193
	Tularemia	UCV-1	MICRO-2	Infectious Disease	69
	Twin Pregnancy	UCV-2	OB/GYN	Obstetrics	52
	Typhoid Fever	UCV-1	MICRO-2	Infectious Disease	70
	Typhoid Fever	UCV-2	IM-2	Infectious Disease	30
U	Ulcerative Colitis	UCV-1	PATHOPHYS-1	Gastroenterology	102
	Ulcerative Colitis	UCV-2	IM-1	Gastroenterology	40
	Umbilical Hernia	MC	SURG	General Surgery	363
	Urate Nephropathy	UCV-1	PATHOPHYS-2	Nephrology/Urology	72
	Ureteral Injury—Iatrogenic	UCV-1	ANAT	General Surgery	37
	Urethritis	UCV-2	ER	Infectious Disease	27
	Urethritis—Nongonococcal	UCV-1	MICRO-2	Infectious Disease	71
	Urinary Tract Infection (UTI)	UCV-1	MICRO-2	Infectious Disease	72
	Urinary Tract Infection (UTI)	UCV-2	IM-2	Infectious Disease	31
	Urticaria	MC	ER	Dermatology	21
	Urticaria	UCV-1	MICRO-1	Dermatology	16
	Uterine Fibroids	UCV-1	PATHOPHYS-3	OB/GYN Gynecology	58
	Uterine Fibroids	UCV-2	OB/GYN	Gynecology	28
	Uterine Leiomyosarcoma	UCV-1	PATHOPHYS-3	Gynecology	59
	Uterine Prolapse with Cystocele	UCV-1	ANAT	Gynecology	40
	Uterine Prolapse with Cystocele	UCV-2	OB/GYN	Gynecology	29
	UTI with Staphylococcus saprophyticus	UCV-1	MICRO-2	Infectious Disease	73
	Uveitis	MC	ER	ENT/Ophthalmology	37
	Uveitis	UCV-1	PATHOPHYS-1	ENT/Ophthalmology	74
V	Vaginismus	UCV-1	BEHAV-SC	Somatoform Disorders	95
	Vaginitis—Atrophic	MC	OB/GYN	Gynecology	285
	Vaginitis—Candidal	UCV-2	OB/GYN	Gynecology	30
	Vaginitis—Trichomonas	UCV-2	OB/GYN	Gynecology	31
	Varicella Zoster (Chickenpox)	UCV-1	MICRO-2	Infectious Disease	74
	Varicella Zoster (Chickenpox)	UCV-2	PED	Infectious Disease	35
	Varicose Veins	MC	SURG	General Surgery	364
	Varicose Veins	UCV-1	ANAT	General Surgery	38
	Vasectomy	UCV-1	ANAT	Nephrology/Urology	48
	Ventricular Fibrillation	UCV-2	ER	Cardiology	6
	Ventricular Flutter	MC	ER	Cardiology	16
	Ventricular Septal Defect	UCV-1	ANAT	Cardiology	8
	Ventricular Septal Defect	UCV-2	PED	Cardiology	3
	Verapamil Side Effects	UCV-1	PHARM	Cardiology	11

	Case Name	SER	BOOK	SubSpecialty	Case Number
	Vertebrobasilar Insufficiency	MC	IM-2	Neurology	205
	Viagra	UCV-1	PHARM	Nephrology/Urology	61
	Vibrio parahaemolyticus Food Poisoning	UCV-1	MICRO-1	Gastroenterology	41
	Vibrio vulnificus Food Poisoning	UCV-1	MICRO-1	Gastroenterology	42
	Visceral Larva Migrans	UCV-1	MICRO-2	Infectious Disease	75
	Vitamin A Deficiency	MC	PED	Endocrinology	309
	Vitamin A Deficiency	UCV-1	BIOCHEM	Endocrinology	32
	Vitamin A Toxicity	MC	IM-2	Dermatology	152
	Vitamin A Toxicity	UCV-1	PHARM	Dermatology	13
	Vitamin B_1 Deficiency (Beriberi)	UCV-1	BIOCHEM	Endocrinology	33
	Vitamin B_3 Deficiency (Pellagra)	UCV-1	BIOCHEM	Endocrinology	34
	Vitamin C Deficiency (Scurvy)	UCV-1	BIOCHEM	Endocrinology	35
	Vitamin K Deficiency	UCV-1	BIOCHEM	Endocrinology	36
	Vitiligo	MC	IM-2	Dermatology	153
	Vitiligo	UCV-1	PATHOPHYS-1	Dermatology	48
	Vitreous Hemorrhage	MC	ER	ENT/Ophthalmology	44
	von Gierke's Disease	UCV-1	BIOCHEM	Genetics	73
	von Gierke's Disease	UCV-2	PED	Genetics	15
	von Hippel–Lindau Disease	UCV-1	PATHOPHYS-3	Neurology	35
	von Hippel–Lindau Disease	UCV-2	NEURO	Neurology	50
	von Willebrand's Disease	UCV-1	PATHOPHYS-2	Hematology/Oncology	41
	von Willebrand's Disease	UCV-2	PED	Hematology/Oncology	22
	Vulvar Carcinoma	UCV-1	PATHOPHYS-3	Gynecology	60
	Vulvar Carcinoma	UCV-2	OB/GYN	Gynecology	32
	Vulvar Leukoplakia	MC	OB/GYN	Gynecology	286
	Vulvar Leukoplakia	UCV-1	PATHOPHYS-3	Gynecology	61
	Vulvar Malignant Melanoma	UCV-1	PATHOPHYS-3	OB/GYN Gynecology	62
W	Waldenström's Macroglobulinemia	MC	IM-1	Hematology/Oncology	130
	Waldenström's Macroglobulinemia	UCV-1	PATHOPHYS-2	Hematology/Oncology	42
	Wallenberg's Syndrome	UCV-1	ANAT	Neurology	73
	Warfarin Interactions	UCV-1	PHARM	Hematology/Oncology	41
	Warfarin Toxicity	UCV-1	PHARM	Hematology/Oncology	42
	Warfarin Toxicity	UCV-2	ER	Hematology/Oncology	24
	Wegener's Granulomatosis	UCV-1	PATHOPHYS-3	Rheumatology	96
	Wegener's Granulomatosis	UCV-2	IM-2	Rheumatology	57
	Wernicke–Korsakoff Syndrome	UCV-1	BIOCHEM	Neurology	86
	Wernicke–Korsakoff Syndrome	UCV-2	PSYCH	Neurology	3
	Whipple's Disease	MC	IM-1	Gastroenterology	111

	Case Name	SER	BOOK	SubSpecialty	Case Number
	Whipple's Disease	UCV-1	MICRO-1	Gastroenterology	43
	Whooping Cough	MC	PED	Infectious Disease	327
	Whooping Cough	UCV-1	MICRO-2	Infectious Disease	76
	Wilms' Tumor	UCV-1	PATHOPHYS-2	Nephrology/Urology	73
	Wilms' Tumor	UCV-2	PED	Nephrology/Urology	48
	Wilson's Disease	UCV-1	BIOCHEM	Gastroenterology	41
	Wilson's Disease	UCV-2	PED	Gastroenterology	9
	Wiskott–Aldrich Syndrome	UCV-1	PATHOPHYS-2	Hematology/Oncology	43
	Wiskott–Aldrich Syndrome	UCV-2	PED	Hematology/Oncology	23
	Withholding Treatment	UCV-2	PSYCH	Ethics	35
	Wolff–Parkinson–White Syndrome	UCV-1	PATHOPHYS-1	Cardiology	28
	Wolff–Parkinson–White Syndrome	UCV-2	IM-1	Cardiology	15
	Wrist—Barton's Fracture	MC	SURG	Orthopedics	378
	Wrist—Carpal Tunnel Syndrome	UCV-1	ANAT	Orthopedics	98
	Wrist—Colles' Fracture	UCV-2	SURG	Orthopedics	49
	Wrist—Scaphoid Fracture	MC	SURG	Orthopedics	379
	Wrist—Scaphoid Fracture	UCV-1	ANAT	Orthopedics	99
	Wrist Slash Injury	UCV-1	ANAT	Orthopedics	100
X	Xeroderma Pigmentosum	UCV-1	BIOCHEM	Genetics	74
	X-Linked Hypogammaglobulinemia	UCV-1	MICRO-2	Immunology	6
Y	Yaws	UCV-1	MICRO-2	Infectious Disease	77
	Yellow Fever	UCV-1	MICRO-2	Infectious Disease	78
	Yersinia Enterocolitis	UCV-1	MICRO-1	Gastroenterology	44
Z	Zidovudine Toxicity	UCV-1	PHARM	Infectious Disease	56
	Zollinger–Ellison Syndrome	MC	IM-1	Gastroenterology	112
	Zollinger–Ellison Syndrome	UCV-1	PATHOPHYS-1	Gastroenterology	103